EMERGENCIES IN ENDODONTICS

Dr. Aishwarya Patil & Dr. Priyanka Zinge

notionpress.com

INDIA • SINGAPORE • MALAYSIA

ISBN
Paperback 979-8-90342-753-6
Hardcase 979-8-90342-754-3

CONTENTS

ACKNOWLEDGEMENT

We express our profound gratitude to **Dr. Suresh Bhosale, Hon'ble Chancellor, Krishna Vishwa Vidyapeeth (Deemed to be University),** for their guidance, inspiration, and for providing a strong academic foundation that made this work possible.

We would also like to express our deepest gratitude to our families for their constant encouragement, unconditional support, and unwavering belief in us throughout this journey.

ABOUT THE AUTHORS

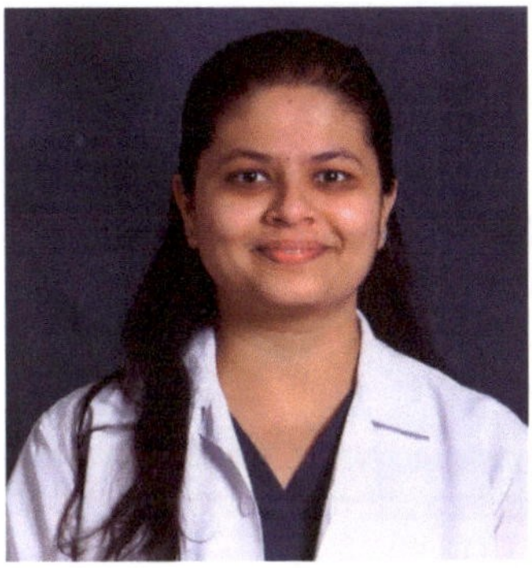

Dr. Aishwarya Patil

Dr. Aishwarya Patil is a Third-Year Postgraduate Student in the Department of Conservative Dentistry and Endodontics at the School of Dental Sciences, Krishna Vishwa Vidyapeeth (Deemed-to-be University), Karad. She completed her Bachelor of Dental Surgery (BDS) from the School of Dental Sciences, Karad.

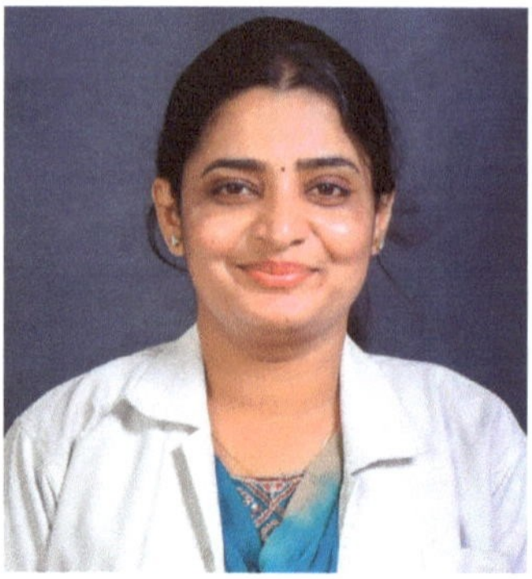

Dr. Priyanka zinge

Dr. Priynka Zinge is an Associate Professor, PG Guide, and PhD Scholar in the Department of Conservative Dentistry and Endodontics, School of Dental Sciences, Krishna Vishwa Vidyapeeth, Karad, Maharashtra.

She received her BDS degree from Bharati Vidyapeeth Dental College, Sangli (BVDU), and her MDS degree from PMNM Dental College, Bagalkot (RGUHS University) in 2014 and 2018, respectively.

She has presented several research and clinical papers at various conferences and has entitled multiple research articles, copyrights, as well as patents.

INTRODUCTION

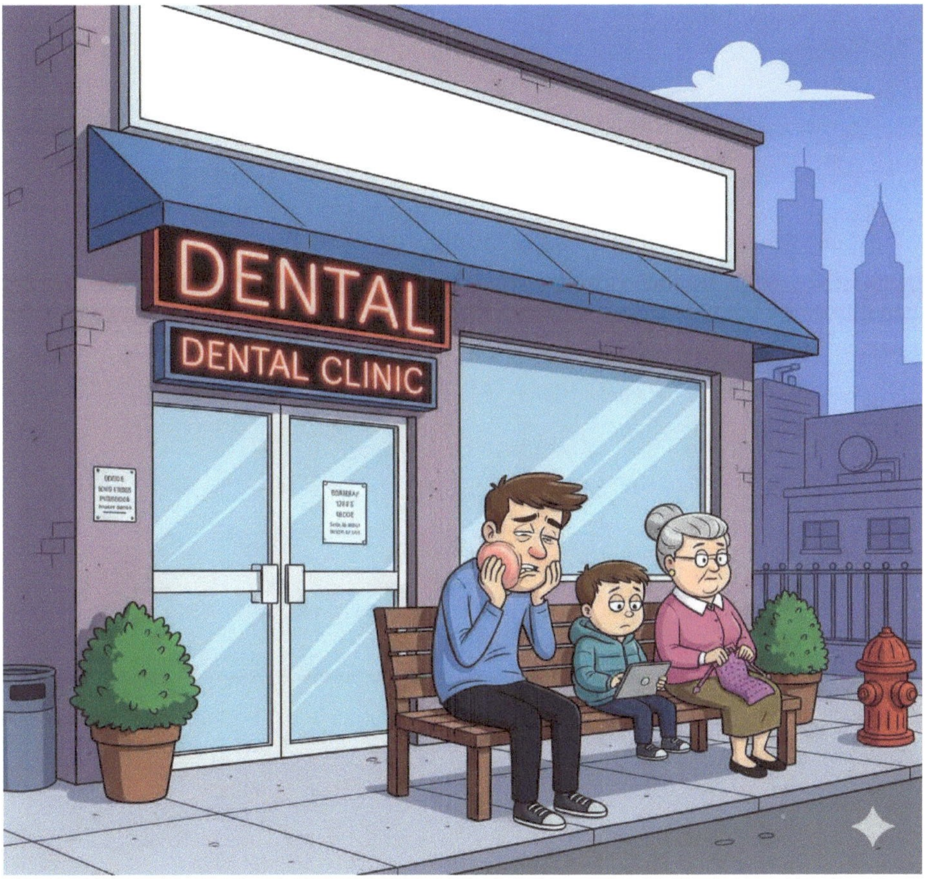

INTRODUCTION

Imagine you are enjoying a scrumptious dinner and are suddenly greeted by unwelcome guests and your planned personal schedule goes for a toss. This is exactly what endodontic emergencies are – unwelcome guests that need to be dealt with diligently. A dentist is often judged by the promptness with which he caters to a patient in pain and provides pain relief.

Endodontic emergencies demand precise diagnosis and skilled management, drawing on multiple aspects of endodontic expertise. Any lapse, whether in diagnosis or treatment, can worsen the patient's condition instead of relieving their pain. The dentist must know pain mechanisms, patient management, diagnosis, anesthesia, therapeutics, and appropriate treatment measures for both hard and soft tissues.

Fun fact: Around 90% patients seeking emergency dental treatment suffer from pulpal or periapical disease.[1]

What is an endodontic emergency?

"An endodontic emergency can be defined as occurring when a patient has pain associated with inflammation of the pulp and/ or periradicular tissues, or when there is pain (with or without swelling) caused by infection of the root canal system and/or the periradicular tissues".[2]

Endodontic emergencies concern patients, dentists, and staff alike. Pain or swelling can arise before, during, or after root canal treatment, often resulting from irritants that trigger intense inflammation in the pulp and periradicular tissues.[2]root canal and periradicular tissues. They may occur before endodontic treatment has been started, between appointments when treatment is being performed over multiple visits, or after endodontic treatment has been completed. In the latter situation, the emergency may be very soon after the treatment or it may occur many years later, in which case it is usually a new disease process as a result of the root canal system becoming infected. An emergency can be a stressful situation for both the patient and the dentist (or endodontist Various factors such as age, gender and tooth type contribute to the emergence of endodontic emergencies; however, the cause-and-effect relationships remain inconclusive.[3,4]

The role of bacteria and their by-products in dental emergencies is well recognized. Bacteria are key contributors to the development of pulpal and periradicular diseases. Mixed bacterial flora, particularly Gram-negative anaerobes are often associated with the clinical signs and symptoms of periradicular infections. Additionally, bacterial by-products such as collagenase, chondroitinase, and hyaluronidase, commonly found in infected root canals, have been associated with the presence of these clinical symptoms.[5]

Clinicians often regard procedural errors, such as instrument separation, perforations, overfilling, underfilling, or ledge formation as the primary causes of endodontic failure. However, these technical mishaps alone rarely compromise treatment success unless accompanied by infection. Scientific evidence shows that even well-executed endodontic treatments may fail due to other contributing factors, including microbial causes (intraradicular and extraradicular infections) and nonmicrobial causes, which may be either intrinsic or extrinsic in nature.[6]

The origin of all pain is inflammation and the inflammatory response.[7] The aim of emergency endodontic treatment is to relieve pain and control any inflammation or infection that may be present. Although insufficient time may prevent ideal treatment from being carried out, the procedures followed should not prejudice any final treatment plan.[3]

Emergency Versus Urgency

It is essential to differentiate between a true emergency from a less critical urgency, irrespective whether occurring before treatment, between appointments, or after obturation. A true emergency is a condition that demands immediate diagnosis and treatment, the patient requires an unscheduled visit that cannot be postponed due to the severity of the problem. In contrast, an urgency represents a milder situation where the appointment can be scheduled at a mutually convenient time for the patient and the dentist.

According to Mahmoud Torabinejad et al. (2021)[8], key questions often asked over the phone can help assess the severity of the problem:

1. **Does the problem interfere with sleeping, eating, working, concentrating, or daily activities?** (A true emergency significantly affects the patient's comfort or quality of life.)
2. **How long has the problem persisted?** (True emergencies typically develop and become severe within a few hours to two days.)
3. **Have you taken any pain medication, and was it effective?** (Pain from a true emergency is usually not relieved by analgesics.)

A positive response to these questions indicates a true emergency requiring prompt management.

The aim of this review is to discuss the approaches for diagnosis and treatment planning of various categories of emergencies. It includes a review of etiologic factors and details of a systematic approach in identifying diagnosing and treating the offending cause.

HISTORY

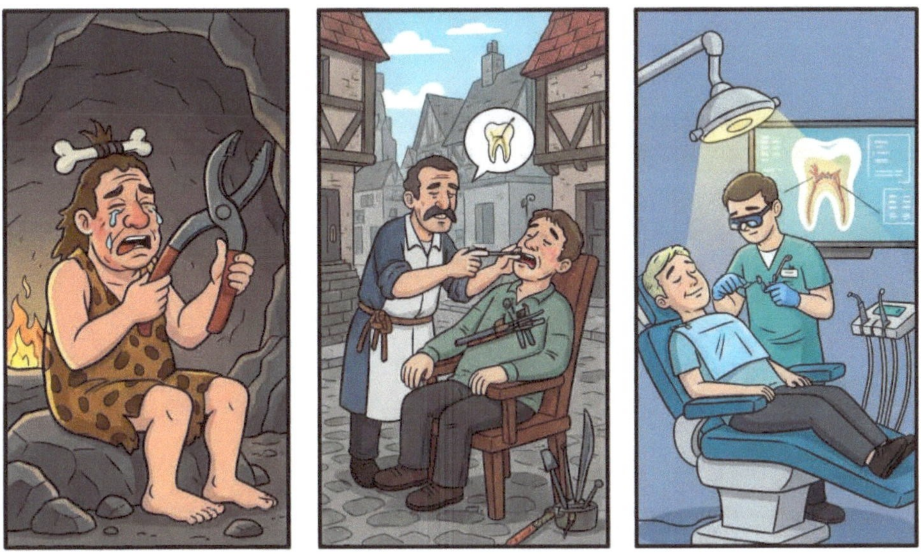

HISTORY

1. Ancient Origins

The history of endodontic emergencies can be traced back to early civilizations where dental pain was among the most distressing ailments.

- Ancient Mesopotamian cuneiform tablets (2000 BC) attributed toothache to the presence of a "**tooth worm**". Egyptian and Babylonian records describe similar beliefs, and treatment usually consisted of herbal applications or charms, with extraction as the only definitive solution.[9]
- In traditional Chinese medicine, toothache was regarded as a **systemic imbalance** and treated with acupuncture and topical herbal remedies.[4]
- Greek and Roman physicians described painful oral swellings resembling **abscesses**.
- Hippocrates and Galen recommended **cautery or extraction for relief**, recognizing that untreated infection could threaten general health.
- However, during the medieval period, emergency dental care remained primitive and was largely confined to extraction performed by barbers or lay practitioners.[9]

  They weren't wrong… were they?

  We now know that oral health affects overall health.

2. Renaissance and Early Modern Period (16th–18th Century)

The Renaissance revived interest in anatomy and oral disease.

- Andreas Vesalius (1543) documented oral anatomy in **De Humani Corporis Fabrica**, offering better understanding of dental structures.
- The true landmark was Pierre Fauchard's **Le Chirurgien Dentiste** (1728), where pulp pathology was described in detail. Fauchard suggested pulp extirpation as an alternative to extraction in acute emergencies.

This marked the beginning of attempts to preserve teeth affected by endodontic disease rather than removing them.[9]

3. The 19th Century: Scientific Advancements

The 19th century brought significant innovations that shaped modern endodontic emergency management:

- **Gutta-percha (1847):** Edwin Truman introduced gutta-percha as a root canal filling material, providing reliable obturation and stabilization of emergency cases.[9]
- **Anesthesia:** The introduction of nitrous oxide (Horace Wells, 1844) and ether anesthesia (William Morton, 1846) allowed invasive procedures such as pulpotomy and pulpectomy to be performed with reduced patient suffering.[4]
- **Antisepsis:** Lister's principles of antiseptic surgery influenced dental practice, and medicaments such as phenol were introduced into pulp chambers for emergency pain relief.[9]
- **Radiography:** Wilhelm Roentgen's discovery of X-rays in 1895 enabled visualization of periapical pathology and traumatic fractures, revolutionizing diagnosis in acute emergencies.[10]

4. Early 20th Century: Microbiology and Standardization

- The role of bacteria in pulpal and periapical pathology was confirmed in the early 20th century, shifting focus from symptomatic treatment to microbiological control.
- Louis I. Grossman played a pivotal role in **standardizing endodontic practice** through successive editions of Endodontic Practice (final 11th edition, 1992), where he outlined protocols for managing irreversible pulpitis, acute apical abscesses, and flare-ups.[9]
- In 1943, the establishment of the **American Association of Endodontists (AAE)** gave the specialty institutional recognition, with structured guidelines for emergency procedures such as incision and drainage, pulpotomy, and pulpectomy. [11]

5. Mid 20th Century: Antibiotics and Medicaments

- The discovery and widespread use of **penicillin** in the 1940s significantly reduced morbidity and mortality associated with odontogenic infections, such as Ludwig's angina and cavernous sinus thrombosis.[4]
- **Calcium hydroxide**, introduced in the same period, became the gold-standard intracanal medicament due to its antibacterial and tissue-dissolving properties.[9]
- Emergency endodontic care now combined **mechanical canal debridement with intracanal medicaments and antibiotics** when systemic involvement was present.[4]

6. Late 20th Century: Classification and Diagnostic Precision

By the latter half of the 20th century, endodontic emergencies were systematically classified. Hargreaves and Berman[12] describe them as:

- Symptomatic irreversible pulpitis
- Symptomatic apical periodontitis

- Acute apical abscess
- Phoenix abscess (flare-up during or after treatment)

These classifications provided diagnostic clarity and guided treatment decisions. Improved diagnostic aids, including electric pulp testing and refined radiographic techniques, enhanced the accuracy of emergency management.[12]

7. 21st Century: Evidence-Based and Regenerative Approaches

In modern practice, endodontic emergency management emphasizes minimally invasive and biologically driven interventions:

- **Advanced imaging:** Digital radiography and cone-beam computed tomography (CBCT) allow three-dimensional visualization of periapical lesions and trauma.[13]
- **Antibiotic stewardship:** Contemporary studies show general practitioners often overprescribe antibiotics compared with specialists, leading to stewardship campaigns restricting use to cases with systemic involvement.[14]
- **Dental education:** Simulation models, including 3D-printed case scenarios, are used to train students in managing endodontic emergencies before clinical exposure.[13]
- **Vital pulp therapy:** Surveys reveal students increasingly prefer pulp vitality tests and conservative pulpotomy over extraction for acute pain.[15]
- **Regenerative protocols:** For immature permanent teeth with pulp necrosis due to trauma, regenerative endodontic procedures and apexification are recommended as first-line treatments.[16]

Thus, the history of endodontic emergencies represents a continuous evolution from extraction-based interventions to highly sophisticated, evidence-based, and biologically oriented approaches.

DEFINITION OF ENDODONTIC EMERGENCIES

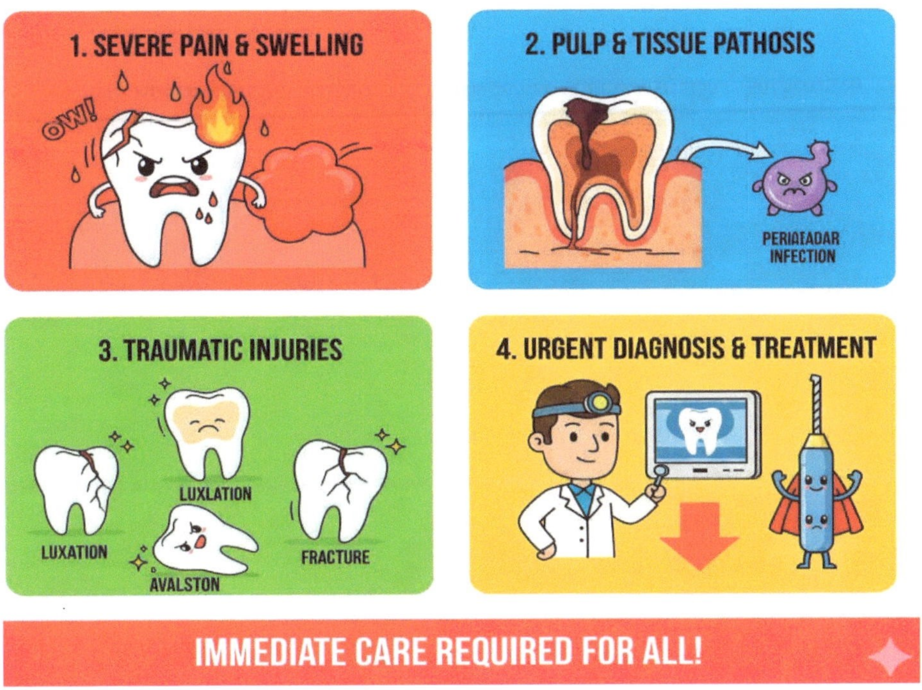

DEFINITION OF ENDODONTIC EMERGENCIES

Definition

"Endodontic emergencies are usually associated with pain and/or swelling and require immediate diagnosis and treatment. These emergencies are caused by pathosis in the pulp or periradicular tissues. They also include severe traumatic injuries that result in luxation, avulsion, or fractures of the hard tissues." (Principles and practice of endodontics, Mahmoud Torabinejad 3rd ed[8])

"An endodontic emergency is defined as pain and/or swelling caused by inflammation or infection of the pulp and/or periradicular tissues necessitating an emergency visit to the dentist for immediate treatment." (Grossman's Endodontic practice 13th ed[9])

"An endodontic emergency is defined as pain or swelling caused by various stages of inflammation or infection of the pulpal or periapical tissues." (Cohen 11th ed[12])

CLASSIFICATION OF ENDODONTIC EMERGENCIES

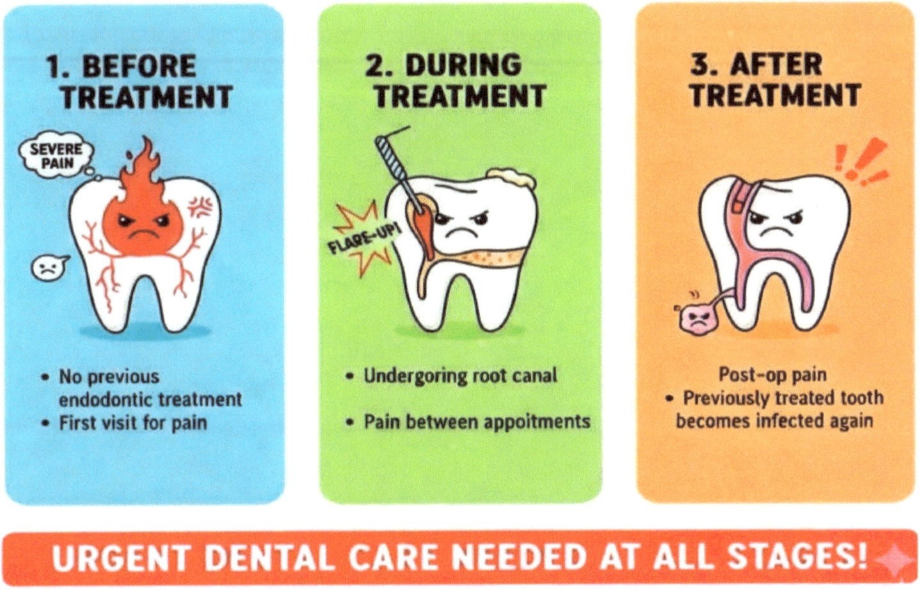

CLASSIFICATION OF ENDODONTIC EMERGENCIES

Endodontic emergencies have been classified in various ways by several authors, but a common system has been to consider endodontic emergencies in relation to the timing of root canal treatment.[2]

Endodontic emergencies that occur

1. **Prior to endodontic treatment:** teeth that have not had any previous endodontic treatment;
2. **During endodontic treatment:** (usually root canal treatment or root canal re-treatment): teeth undergoing treatment over >1 appointment; these emergencies are often referred to as a "flare-up" and
3. **After endodontic treatment:** post-operative pain following the root canal filling stage of treatment or teeth that have had previous root canal treatment at some time in the past and have become infected again which has led to acute apical periodontitis or an acute apical abscess.

Classification of Endodontic Emergencies (According to P Carrotte)[17]

Table 3.1

Type	Pre- treatment	Intra-treatment	Post-endodontic
Definition	Patient comes to the clinician for first time with pain, swelling or injury	Emergency occurring during endodontic treatment	Emergency occurring after completion of endodontic treatment
Conditions	▪ Hot tooth ▪ Dentin hypersensitivity ▪ Acute reversible pulpitis ▪ Acute irreversible pulpitis ▪ Acute apical periodontitis ▪ Acute periapical abscess ▪ Traumatic injury ▪ Cracked tooth syndrome	▪ Mid treatment flare-up ▪ Exposure of pulp ▪ Fracture of tooth ▪ Recently placed restoration ▪ Periodontal treatment ▪ Hypochlorite accident ▪ Tissue emphysema	▪ Overextended obturation ▪ Under obturation ▪ Vertical root fracture

According To Louis I. Grossman 1974[9]

1. Acute Conditions

a. Reversible pulpitis

b. Irreversible pulpitis.

c. Alveolar abscess.

d. Periodontal abscess

2. **Emergencies During Treatment**
3. **Fractures of crown and/or root**
4. **Avulsed tooth**
5. **Referred pain**

According to surveys taken among endodontists in 1977, 1990 and 2009 there are seven clinical presentations of endodontic emergencies[12]

1. Irreversible pulpitis and normal periapex
2. Irreversible pulpitis and acute apical periodontitis
3. Necrotic pulp with acute apical periodontitis, with no swelling
4. Necrotic pulp, fluctuant swelling, with drainage
5. Necrotic pulp, fluctuant swelling, with no drainage
6. Necrotic pulp, diffuse facial swelling, with drainage through canals
7. Necrotic pulp, diffuse facial swelling, with no drainage.

According to Torabinejad principles and practice of endodontics, 3rd edition[8]

1. Pretreatment emergency

These are situations in which the patient is seen initially with severe pain and/or swelling.

2. Interappointment and postobturation emergency

Also referred to as the "flare-up," this problem occurs after an endodontic appointment. Although an upsetting event, this is easier to manage because the offending tooth has already been identified and a diagnosis has been previously established.

DIAGNOSIS OF ENDODONTIC EMERGENCIES

1. DIAGOSTIC STEPS

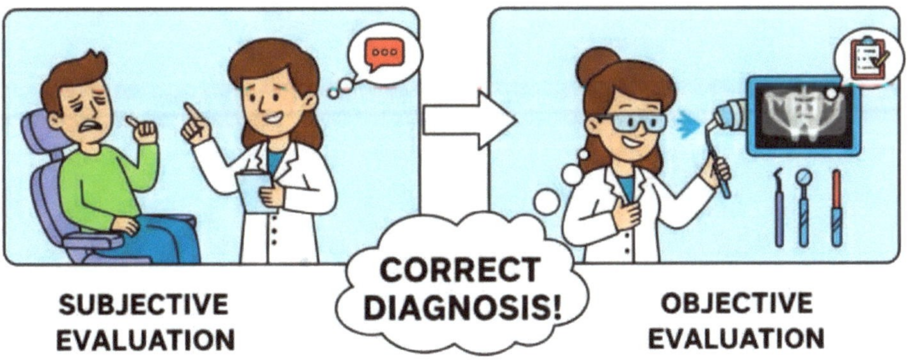
SUBJECTIVE EVALUATION
CORRECT DIAGNOSIS!
OBJECTIVE EVALUATION

2. ROLES IN PAIN MANAGEMENT

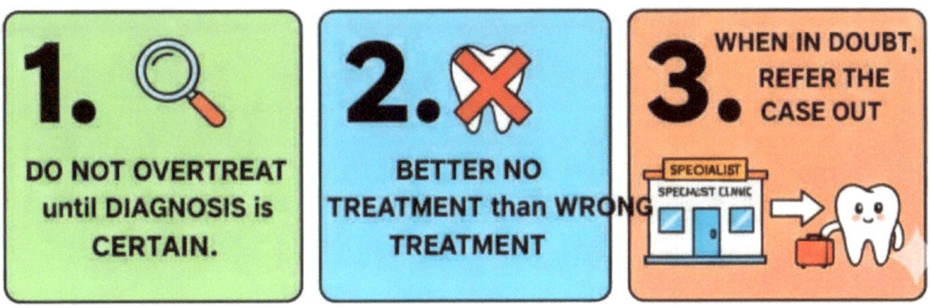
1.
DO NOT OVERTREAT until DIAGNOSIS is CERTAIN.
2.
BETTER NO TREATMENT than WRONG TREATMENT
3.
WHEN IN DOUBT, REFER THE CASE OUT
SPECIALIST

DIAGNOSIS OF ENDODONTIC EMERGENCIES

Every dentist has faced it : a patient walking in with severe tooth pain demanding immediate relief. Managing such an endodontic emergency calls for a blend of sharp diagnostic skills, sound knowledge of clinical pharmacology, and expertise in endodontic procedures. When applied correctly, these skills enable the clinician to provide prompt and effective care, restoring comfort and trust in a single visit.

Diagnosis

The first step in identifying the cause involves understanding the patient's perception of the problem (**subjective evaluation**), followed by performing appropriate clinical tests (**objective evaluation**) to reproduce and **correlate** with the patient's reported pain symptoms.[18] Correct diagnosis of the emergency patient's orofacial signs and symptoms is a prerequisite for their proper management.[9]

There are 3 roles in management of pain in emergency:

1. Do not over treat until you are certain from the diagnosis.
2. It is better to provide no treatment than to provide wrong treatment.
3. When you are in doubt refer the case out.

Five objective clinical tests need to be performed in a patient's endodontic diagnostic evaluation:[18]

1. Cold test, electric pulp tester (EPT) and/or heat tests for pulp vitality
2. Percussion testing to determine the status of the periodontal ligament.
3. Palpation testing to evaluate the gingival tissue and cortical and trabecular bone for infection or inflammation.
4. Periodontal examination that includes probing and tooth mobility evaluation.
5. Radiographic examination of current periapical and bitewing films, along with CBCT (cone-beam computed tomography) when indicated.

Differential Diagnosis[18]

Orofacial signs and symptoms may arise from non-odontogenic etiologies, and because such pathologic entities may co-exist with confirmed endodontic and periodontal abnormalities, differential diagnosis of non-dental origin should always be considered whenever the dentist evaluates symptoms for probable cause.

Non-odontogenic causes of orofacial symptoms can be classified into several categories:

1. Organic
2. Functional
3. Vascular
4. Neuralgic
5. Psychogenic

It should be emphasized that the main purpose of categorizing the various non-dentoalveolar conditions is to facilitate the eventual referral of the patient to the appropriate medical of dental specialist.

1. Organic Disorder/Alteration In The Structure Of Body Organ Adapted To Specific Function

e.g.: Non-dental mandibular paresthesia is most suggestive of an impinging tumor; maxillary and facial paresthesia not attributable to dental origin is probably due to maxillary sinus disease

The fact that the alveolar process of the maxillary posterior teeth also forms the inferior portion of maxillary sinus help to explain this observation.

2. Functional Disorder

Functional disorders affect the normal performance of an organ or tissue without apparent organic or structural changes. e.g.: (MPDS) myofascial pain-dysfunction syndrome involving TMJ region.

Symptoms:

i. Severe emotional stress

ii. Clenching and bruxism

iii. Occlusal disharmonies

3. Vascular Pain Syndromes

e.g. Migraine due to dilation of extra cranial arteries, usually evoked by psychologic factors characterized by post ocular pain, nausea, vomiting.

4. Neuralgic Disorder

e.g. Trigeminal neuralgia is of a primary significance to the dentist because it involves the 5th cranial nerve.

Characteristics of trigeminal neuralgia

- Sharp, shooting or stabbing attack similar to an electro shock.
- Sudden recurrent, extremely intense and short episodes
- Main feature: Presence of a trigger zone around the mouth, face or throat provoking stimuli may include light touch, talking, chewing, swallowing, washing the face and blowing the nose.

Differential diagnosis: dental disorders (e.g. irreversible pulpitis, cracked tooth).

5. Psychogenic Disorder

e.g. Psychogenic facial pain and headache may result from states of dejection and mental depression.

If the chief complaint has been positively identified as an endodontic problem and the location has been precisely determined, inform the patient regarding pertinent examination finding (e.g.: pre-existing periodontal condition, pulpal status, extent of alveolar involvement, restorative considerations) recommended treatment plan, alternative approaches, risks and prognosis.

PRE-OPERATIVE ENDODONTIC EMERGENCIES

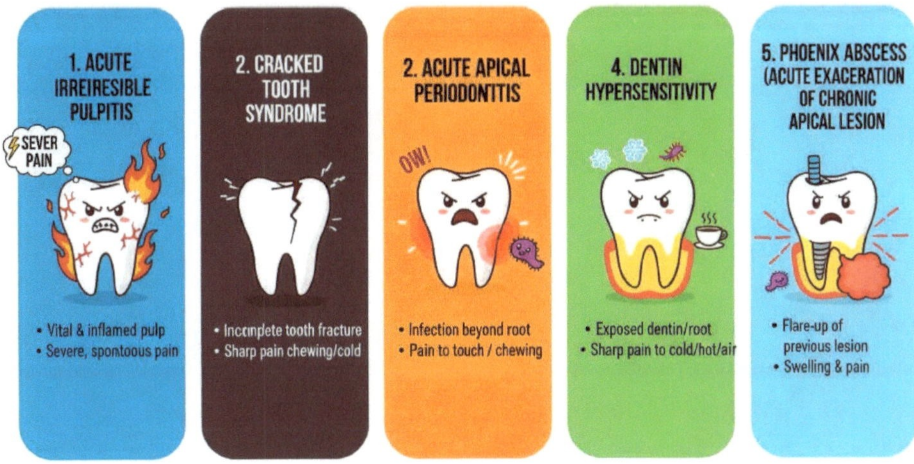

PRE-OPERATIVE ENDODONTIC EMERGENCIES

Pre-operative endodontic emergencies include myriad clinical situations in which the pulp is either vital and inflamed, as in cases of acute irreversible pulpitis, or has undergone partial or complete necrosis.

- They may also involve conditions where bacterial products have extended beyond the root canal system, eliciting inflammation of the periodontal ligament, as seen in acute apical periodontitis.

Such emergencies typically present with severe pain, localized or diffuse swelling, and significant patient distress, often prompting urgent dental consultation. In these situations, the inflammatory response is usually initiated by microbial invasion, most often due to caries, trauma, or restorative procedures, which allows microorganisms and their by-products to penetrate the pulp and periapical tissues.[19]

If left untreated: Infection may progress beyond the confines of the apical foramen → invasion of adjacent alveolar bone and soft tissues → acute alveolar abscess characterized by pain, swelling, tenderness, and possible systemic involvement such as fever and lymphadenopathy.[19]

Accurate diagnosis is essential in such cases

A thorough case history should include assessment of:

- Subjective findings (patient history, chief complaint, pain characteristics)
- Objective assessments (clinical tests and radiographic evaluation)
- Patient's description of the onset, duration, nature, and aggravating or relieving factors of pain (often pivotal in differentiating between pulpal, periapical, and periodontal etiologies)

Understanding the stage of pulpal and periapical pathosis influences the choice of emergency intervention whether pulp extirpation, incision and drainage, occlusal reduction, or pharmacologic management. Preoperative emergencies thus represent a crucial phase in endodontic care, where timely and accurate intervention can significantly improve prognosis and patient comfort while preventing progression to more severe odontogenic infections.

5.1 DENTIN HYPERSENSITIVITY

Dentine sensitivity (DS) or dentinal hypersensitivity (DH) is one of the commonly encountered clinical problems. It is clinically described as an exaggerated response to a stimulus to exposed dentine, regardless of its location.

True hypersensitivity can develop due to pulpal inflammation, presenting with clinical features of irreversible pulpitis i.e., severe and persistent pain, as compared with typical short sharp pain of DH.[20]

Definition

"Dentine hypersensitivity is characterized by short, sharp pain arising from exposed dentine in response to stimuli, typically thermal, evaporative, tactile, osmotic or chemical and which cannot be ascribed to any other dental defect or pathology"

International workshop on DH, 1997 [21]

Some facts

- **Prevalence**: 4-74% in different groups.[20]
- **Most frequently affected teeth**: permanent canines and premolars.[22]
- **Frequently affected sites**: Buccal cervical regions.[22]
- **Age**: The symptom can present at any age, but the majority of individuals range from 20 to 40 years, with a peak in prevalence at the end of the third decade.[22]
- **Gender**: Females >> males, and at a younger mean age, possibly due to more frequent and extensive oral hygiene episodes. The decline in prevalence after age 40 may be due to the levels of secondary and reparative dentine.[22]

Why do we get pain?

Imagine this: A patient sits in your dental chair, wincing the moment a cold burst of air hits their tooth. It's not decay, not a crack — just that familiar sharp, fleeting pain that makes them flinch. Within seconds, it's gone, but the memory lingers.

Pain, after all, isn't just a physical sensation. It's an unpleasant sensory and emotional experience linked to actual or potential tissue damage ; a definition that perfectly captures the complexity of managing pain in dental practice.[23]

All individuals experience pain differently; thresholds vary, and so do reactions. That's what makes dentine hypersensitivity such a challenge to evaluate. The pain is subjective; what feels like a mild twinge to one person can be unbearable to another. Typically, dentine hypersensitivity presents as a rapid-onset, sharp pain triggered by a thermal, tactile, or osmotic stimulus, disappearing as quickly as it appears. Occasionally, though, the discomfort lingers, transforming into a dull, throbbing ache that persists long after the stimulus is gone.[20]

Three major mechanisms of dentinal sensitivity have been proposed in the literature

1. Direct innervation theory
2. Odontoblast receptor
3. Fluid movement/hydrodynamic theory

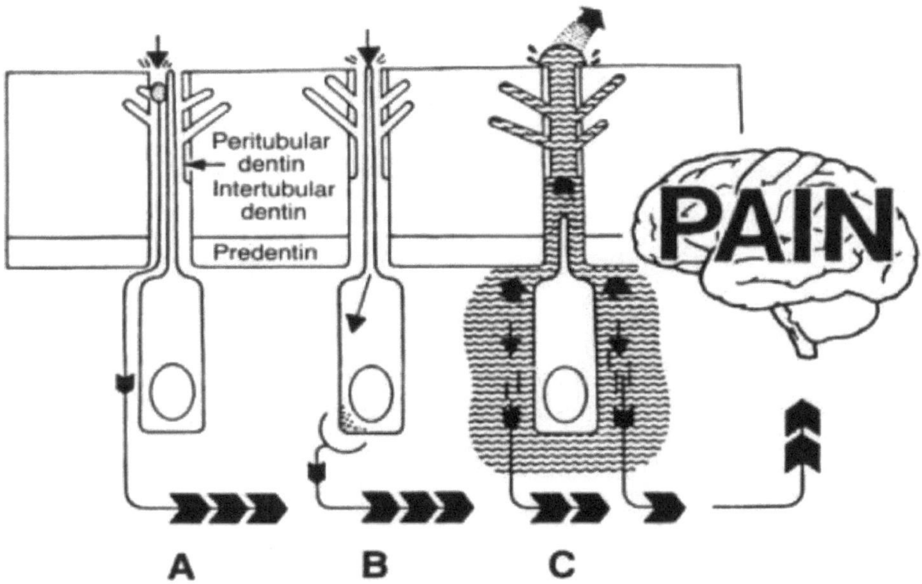

Figure 1: The schematic picture of the propped theories on DH. A. Direct innervation theory B. Odontoblast receptor C. Fluid movement / hydrodynamic theory[24]

Direct Innervation Theory[20, 25]

According to this theory, nerve endings penetrate dentine and extend to the dentino-enamel junction. Direct mechanical stimulation of these nerves will initiate an action potential. Developmental studies have shown that the plexus of Rashkow and intratubular nerves do not establish themselves until the tooth has erupted; yet, newly erupted tooth is sensitive.

Odontoblast Receptor Theory[20,26]

It states that odontoblasts act as receptors by themselves and relay the signal to a nerve terminal. But studies have shown that odontoblasts are matrix forming cells and hence they are not considered to be excitable cells, and no synapses have been demonstrated between odontoblasts and nerve terminals.

Fluid Movement/Hydrodynamic Theory[20,26,27]

This theory was first reported by Gysi in 1900. It was extensively studied and corroborated by Brannstrom (1964) who proposed that dentinal pain is due to hydrodynamic mechanism, i.e., fluid force. This theory is based on the presence and movement of fluid inside the dentinal tubules. Centrifugal fluid movement activates the nerve endings at the end of dentinal tubules or at the pulp–dentine complex. The response of pulpal nerves is mainly due to Aδ intradentinal afferent fibers, which depends upon the pressure applied, i.e., intensity of stimuli.

Treatment of Dentin Hypersensitivity[28]

The treatment of dentin hypersensitivity is carried out in three lines of treatment.

- First line of treatment – Confirmation of diagnosis
- Second line of treatment – Consider etiology and behavior.
- Third line of treatment – Management strategies.

First Line of Treatment - Confirmation of Diagnosis

Several dental conditions can give rise to similar pain symptoms of DH. Therefore, the first line of treatment strategy for DH is to reach a definitive diagnosis through elimination of the following conditions:

- Cracked tooth syndrome, often in heavily restored teeth.
- Incorrect placement of dentine adhesives leading to nano leakage.
- Fractured restorations and incorrectly placed dentine pins.
- Inappropriate application of various medicaments during cavity floor preparation.
- Inappropriately contoured restorations so the tooth is in traumatic occlusion.

- Palatogingival groove and other enamel invaginations and defects.
- Chipped teeth causing exposed dentine.
- Vital tooth bleach
- Pulpal response to caries and recent restorative treatment.

Clinical examination for the diagnosis of DH would include objective assessments such as:

- Mechanical/tactile stimuli, for example running a sharp explorer over the area of the exposed dentine.
- Thermal and evaporative stimuli, such as a blast of cold air from the triple syringe.
- For DH to occur, dentin must be exposed, and some tubules need to be patent throughout their length from the oral environment to the pulp. In most sufferers, exposed dentine is clearly visible.
- If the pain persists after all other pathology is diagnosed and treated, then the diagnosis of DH can be confirmed and the second line of treatment strategy can be started.

Second Line of Treatment – Consider Etiology and Behavior

The etiology of dentin hypersensitivity has two components:

- Dentine needs to become exposed (lesion localization)
- Tubules need to be widely open and patent throughout their length (lesion initiation).

Lesion Localization

- Dentin in most young adults is exposed to oral environment, due to loss of cementum and enamel, but clinical experience indicates that only a proportion suffer from DH.

- Any process causing cervical dentin exposure (enamel erosion, gingival recession, or an anatomical defect) and tubular opening (loss of the smear layer which normally occludes tubules in exposed dentine) can lead to tooth sensitivity, suggesting a **multifactorial etiology.**
- Loss of enamel is predominantly a process of erosion (caused by exposure to intrinsic or extrinsic acids) often accompanied by abrasion, attrition or abfraction.
- The buccal cervical lesion with exposed dentine due to enamel loss is most likely due to an individual being susceptible to erosion and an aggressive tooth brushing technique in conjunction with abrasive cleaning agents found in all toothpastes
- When an acid encounters the tooth, not only is there bulk loss of the hard tissue but also softening of the remaining surface. In vitro research has shown that surface softening can extend to 3-5microns, and be susceptible to physical loss after a few brush strokes. So, if the erosive challenge is followed soon after with the abrasive challenge (of toothbrush and toothpaste), the softened hard tissue will be easily removed and has no chance to re-harden.
- The role of toothbrush abrasion alone, with and without toothpaste in tooth surface loss has been studied. A toothbrush alone has no measurable effects on enamel and minimal on dentine if a normal twice-a-day regimen is followed.
- Low-abrasive toothpastes will contribute little to hard tissue loss if used twice a day. However, many DH sufferers will brush their teeth in excess, up to five times a day. For these individuals, instruction is necessary, and a low-abrasive paste should be advocated.

Lesion Initiation

- It involves exposing several widely open dentine tubules.
- Erosive challenges will rapidly remove the smear layer and open the dentine tubules. Classic examples which remove the smear layer in minutes are soft drinks, wine, herbal teas and yoghurt.
- Some mouth rinses of low pH can also remove the smear layer. If individuals are susceptible to erosion, milk and water are the drinks of choice.
- If fruit based or carbonated drinks are consumed then it is the frequency, rather than volume, that is important and this should be limited.
- Consumption of drinks with a straw is preferable so long as the straw directs the fluid stream to the back of the mouth and not directly at any tooth.

Behavior: Preventive Advice

- High-risk individuals for erosion are not easy to identify. Thus, the dental team needs to instigate preventive measures for their patients and be vigilant for the first signs of tooth wear, and then to implement therapeutic regimens.
- Mild DH may be the only indication that tooth wear is occurring.
- Owing to less enamel thickness at the cervical margin, only a few microns of enamel surface loss need to occur for dentine to become exposed.
- This is most likely due to erosion, abrasion and environmental stimuli. Cold wintery weather in temperate climates or the onset of mango season in tropical climates, bring many more complaints of DH.

List of Preventive Factors

- Etiological factors need to be modified to protect and cover the dentine surface to reduce pain symptoms.
- Assess the frequency of consuming erosive drinks and thus the interval in-between
- Take diet history probing for frequency of acid intake in conjunction with a detailed medical history probing for gastric reflux conditions
- Discourage excessive tooth brushing frequency. Suggest twice daily use of a low abrasive toothpaste.
- Avoid activities that may contribute to the process of gingival recession such as aggressive or abusive oral hygiene habits, tongue jewellery, etc.

Third Line of Treatment - Management Strategies

Clinicians often manage dentine hypersensitivity by relying on what has worked in the past, rather than tailoring treatment to the unique etiological and predisposing factors of each patient. However, because the condition is **multifactorial**, a one-size-fits-all approach rarely yields lasting results. **Effective management begins with identifying and addressing the underlying cause**—whether it's enamel wear, gingival recession, or an abrasive oral care routine.

Today, a wide range of products is available, both for professional application and home use, all designed to offer varying degrees of symptom relief. Yet, true success lies not merely in reducing sensitivity, but in understanding why it occurs in the first place.

The two main approaches in the treatment of dentine hypersensitivity are:

- Modification or blocking of pulpal nerve response.
- Alteration of fluid flow in dentinal tubules

Modification or Blocking of Pulpal Nerve Response

A. Chemical methods.

- Potassium ions may reduce interdental nerve excitability by diffusing along the tubules and raising the concentration of local extracellular potassium ions, hence blocking interdental nerve function.
- The Canadian Advisory Board on Dentin Hypersensitivity recommended brushing twice daily with desensitizing toothpaste as the first line of treatment.[29]

B. Physical method-endodontic treatment and extraction

- These methods are permanently effective at stopping pain from dentine hypersensitivity by removing the nerve or tooth.
- These should be of last resort and only after thorough diagnosis in conjunction with full mouth and neuropathic assessments.

Alteration of Fluid Flow in Dentinal Tubules

- Blocking the dentinal tubules should reduce or stop any movement of fluid in the tubule.
- This is accomplished in-clinic using varnishes, dentine bonding agents, composite resins, glass ionomer cements and compomers.
- For the occluding agents to be successful they must resist removal. Occluding materials can be washed from the tubule with day-to-day oral salivary clearance or may be acid labile. Wear can also occur, abrading the surface of, for example, a dentine bonding agent or glass ionomer after a couple of months.

1. Administration of Treatment

Treatment can be administered professionally in the office, or by self-care at home, depending on the severity, extent, and persistence of the pain and the patient's preference. In office and at home treatments are not mutually exclusive and may be used adjunctively.

1.1 Self-Care at Home

- Home treatment usually involves desensitizing toothpastes, is by far the simplest and cheapest method and has been endorsed as the first line of treatment.
- The change in toothpaste formulation requires little effort on the part of the patient to ensure relief of symptoms.
- Regular use is essential for symptom relief and a successful outcome.

  a. **Potassium Salts:** Widely available, often result in an improvement in the patient's perceived symptom of DH.

  b. **Strontium Salts**: Strontium chloride and strontium acetate have been incorporated in toothpastes for many years and are well documented. The effectiveness of the product at reducing symptoms appears to increase with increased usage. The rationale for incorporating strontium salts in toothpastes derives from the ability of the salt to have a considerable affinity for dentine, owing to the high permeability and possibility for absorption into or onto the organic connective tissues and the odontoblast processes.

  c. **Oxalates:** Oxalates are thought to occlude tubules by reacting with calcium ions in the dentinal fluid to form insoluble calcium oxalate crystals. While oxalates result in good tubule occlusion, they are acid labile and can be easily washed from the surface of dentine.

  d. **Fluorides:** Various fluoride compounds have been documented for the treatment of dentine hypersensitivity; these include sodium fluoride, sodium silico-fluoride, stannous fluoride and sodium monofluorophosphate. Fluorides may mechanically block the tubules. There are specifically designed mouthwashes and toothpastes for high fluoride uptake which clinically have met with good success.

1.2 Professionally Applied Products

A wide range of commercially available products are available for professional treatment when at-home products have been unsuccessful.

a. **Varnishes and Precipitants:** This approach reduces pain of DH for as long as the agent remains on/in the tubule. Professionally applied sodium fluoride and oxalates have been administered with equivocal efficacy.

b. **Restorative Materials:** Glass ionomer, resin-reinforced glass ionomer/compomers, adhesive resin primers and adhesive resin bonding systems have been used successfully for the treatment of DH. Treatment can be problematic if there has been little tissue loss and over-contouring and inadequate margins can lead to plaque-retentive sites and gingival inflammation. Cavity varnish can give temporary relief of symptoms when applied in a thin film on open dentinal tubules. However, the smear layer must be modified or removed before application, to occlude the tubules and be stable to acidic attack.

c. **Lasers:** Nd: YAG laser irradiation is used for the alleviation of symptoms from DH. They work by coagulation of proteins in the dentinal fluid and hence reduce permeability. They create an amorphous sealed layer on the dentin surface which appears to be due to partial melt down of the surface.

d. **Periodontal Surgery:** Coronally repositioning periodontal flaps to cover areas of exposed dentine has been advocated as a treatment regimen for dentine hypersensitivity. This treatment can be very successful for root coverage but would not be the first choice for treatment for dentine hypersensitivity due to being an invasive procedure and in terms of cost.

In conclusion, managing dentine hypersensitivity often requires a combination of approaches, as the underlying causes can vary widely from one patient to another. Clinicians are encouraged to begin with the **least invasive treatment options**, progressing to professionally applied therapies if symptoms persist. Since dentine hypersensitivity frequently arises in association with **gingival recession or erosive tooth wear**, it is essential to address these **predisposing factors** alongside symptom relief. Only by tackling the root causes can long-term comfort and clinical success be achieved.

Recent Advances in the Management of Dentine Hypersensitivity

In recent years, there has been remarkable progress in the **therapeutic management of dentine hypersensitivity (DH)**, shifting the focus from temporary symptom relief to **long-lasting, biologically integrated solutions**. Modern approaches aim to achieve **durable occlusion of dentinal tubules** and **enhanced remineralization** by leveraging advances in **biomaterials science, nanotechnology, laser therapy, and bioengineering**. These innovative strategies emphasize **sustained bioactive ion release**, improved **acid resistance**, and **seamless compatibility with natural tooth structure**, offering the potential for more predictable and enduring clinical outcomes.

Bioactive Glasses (BAGs)[30]

- Calcium sodium phosphosilicate bioactive glass (commercially available as NovaMin®) has been extensively investigated for DH management.
- On exposure to saliva, the glass undergoes an ion exchange process, releasing calcium, sodium, and phosphate ions, which subsequently precipitate as amorphous calcium phosphate and crystallize into hydroxycarbonate apatite (HCA), a mineral phase chemically similar to dental apatite.

Casein Phosphopeptide–Amorphous Calcium Phosphate (CPP-ACP)[31]

- CPP-ACP, available commercially as GC Tooth Mousse®, is derived from milk casein and functions by stabilizing amorphous calcium phosphate in a bioavailable state, delivering high concentrations of calcium and phosphate ions to the tooth surface.
- This process promotes remineralization and intratubular mineral deposition, leading to reduced hypersensitivity.
- It is contraindicated in individuals with casein or milk protein allergies.

Nano-Hydroxyapatite (nHAp)[32]

- Nano-hydroxyapatite, a biomimetic form of apatite with particle sizes like enamel crystallites, can integrate with demineralized dentin to form a continuous mineral layer.
- Commercial formulations, such as Aclaim® and Apagard®, have demonstrated comparable or superior efficacy to potassium nitrate-based dentifrices in randomized clinical trials over 4–6 weeks. While effective in remineralization and tubule sealing, regular application is essential for maintaining results.

Arginine–Calcium Carbonate Technology[33]

- The combination of arginine and calcium carbonate, as in Colgate Sensitive Pro-Relief®, produces a positively charged layer on the dentine surface, facilitating occlusion of negatively charged dentinal tubules through ionic bonding and deposition of calcium carbonate crystals.
- Immediate pain relief has been observed after a single professional application, with sustained benefits upon continued home use.
- The main limitation lies in the susceptibility of the occluding layer to acid dissolution.

Bioglass-Enhanced Adhesive Restorative Systems[34]

- Incorporating bioactive glass particles into resin-based adhesive systems allows for sustained release of calcium and phosphate ions post-polymerization, promoting intratubular mineralization while providing mechanical sealing.
- These systems have shown potential benefits for restoring cervical lesions associated with DH, although long-term clinical evidence remains limited.

Laser-Activated Bioglass Sealants[35]

- A novel approach involves applying a bioglass slurry to exposed dentin followed by activation with lasers such as Er: YAG or Nd: YAG.
- Laser energy accelerates crystal formation and fusion to dentine, producing a durable occluding layer.

Magnetic Nanobot Technology (Emerging Research)[36]

- An emerging frontier in DH management involves magnetically guided nanorobots composed of calcium silicate bioceramic nanoparticles.
- These "CalBots" are directed into dentinal tubules up to 500 μm deep, where they self-assemble to form permanent occluding plugs.
  - Preclinical studies at the Indian Institute of Science have demonstrated complete tubule sealing and high acid resistance, though clinical trials are awaited.

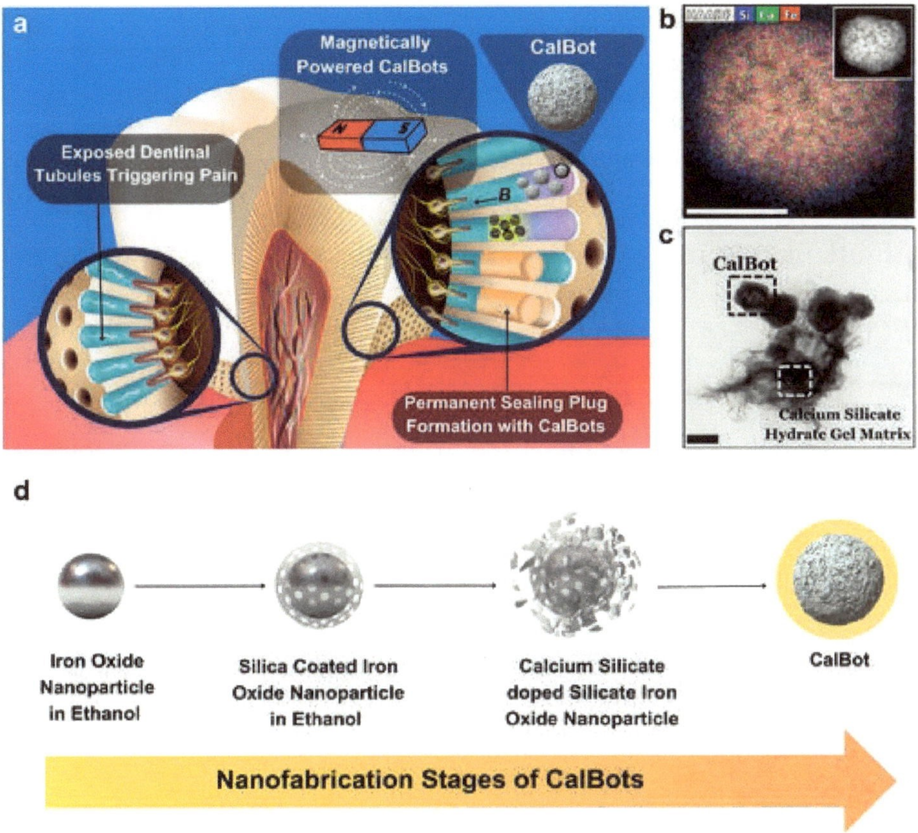

Figure 2: Nanofabrication Stages of CalBots; a) Schematic representation of dental hypersensitivity and the physiology of plug formation inside dentinal tubules using CalBots suspended in CaO gel. b) High-angle annular Dark-Field (HAADF) image of CalBots with elemental analysis. c) Transmission Electron Microscope (TEM) image of CalBots suspended in CaO gel for 30 days showcasing the formation of cohesive calcium silicate hydrate gel matrix amongst neighbouring CalBots. The scale bar represents 200 nm for both the images. d) Schematic representation of nanofabrication stages of CalBots (Adapted from Peddi et al)[36]

5.2 PULPAL DISEASE

A. REVERSIBLE PULPITIS

Definition- Mild to moderate inflammatory condition of the pulp caused by noxious stimuli in which the pulp can return to the uninflamed state following removal of the stimuli. [9]

Etiology

- Trauma blow or from a disturbed occlusal relationship.
- Thermal shock from preparing a cavity with a dull bur or keeping the bur in contact with the tooth for too long without the use of coolant.
- Excessive dehydration of a cavity with alcohol or chloroform.
- Irritation of exposed dentin at the neck of tooth.
- Placement of a fresh amalgam filling in contact with, or occluding, a gold restoration.
- Chemical stimulus as from sweet or sour food stuff.
- Bacteria from caries and anachoresis.

Symptoms

- Sharp pain lasting but moment
- Most often elicited by cold rather than hot food and by cold air.
- Does not occur spontaneously and does not continue when the cause has been removed.

Histopathology

May range from hyperemia to mild to moderate inflammatory changes limited to the area of the involved dentinal tubules, such as dentinal caries.

Microscopically, one may see

- Dilated blood vessel.
- Extravasation of edema fluids.
- Disruption of the odontoblast layer.
- Reparative dentin.
- Acute & Chronic inflammatory cells.

Diagnosis

Diagnosis is based on the symptoms.

- Pain may become chronic. Although each paroxysm may be of short duration, the paroxysms may continue for weeks or even months.
- A tooth with reversible pulpitis reacts normally to percussion, palpation, and mobility, and the periapical tissue is normal on radiographic examination.

Differential diagnosis

1. Irreversible pulpitis : In reversible pulpitis, pain is generally transitory, lasting a matter of seconds whereas in irreversible pulpitis, the pain may last several minutes or longer.

Treatment

1. Best treatment is prevention. - Periodic care to prevent the development of caries. - Early insertion of a filling if a cavity has developed. - Desensitization of tooth neck in case of recession.
2. When reversible pulpitis is present, removal of the noxious stimuli.

3. Once the symptoms have subsided, the tooth should be tested for vitality, to make sure that pulpal necrosis has not occurred.
4. When pain persists despite proper treatment, the pulpal inflammation should be regarded as irreversible, the treatment for which is pulp extirpation.

Prognosis

The prognosis for the pulp is favorable if the irritant is removed early enough; otherwise, the condition may develop into irreversible pulpitis.

B. IRREVERSIBLE PULPITIS

Definition- "It is a persistent inflammatory condition of the pulp, symptomatic or asymptomatic, caused by a noxious stimulus." It has both acute and chronic stages in pulp.[9]

Etiology

- Most common cause of pulpitis is bacterial involvement of pulp through caries
- Chemical, thermal, mechanical injuries of pulp may induce pulp inflammation.
- Reversible pulpitis when left untreated deteriorates into irreversible pulpitis.

Symptoms

- **Pain**
  - Rapid onset caused by sudden temperature change, sweet or acidic food.
  - Remains even after removal of stimulus
  - Spontaneous in nature which is sharp, piercing, intermittent or continuous in nature

- Exacerbated on bending down or lying down due to change in intrapulpal pressure
- Presence of referred pain

In later stages, pain is severe, boring, throbbing in nature which increases with hot stimulus. Pain is so severe that it keeps the patient awake in night. The relief of pain can be simply done by use of cold water. The patient may report dental office with jar of ice water. There is often a history of spontaneous bouts of pain which may last from a few seconds up to several hours.

- When hot or cold fluids are applied, the pain elicited will be prolonged. In the later stages, heat will be more significant; cold may relieve the pain.
- Pain may radiate initially, but once the periodontal ligament has become involved, the patient will be able to locate the tooth.
- The tooth becomes tender to percussion once inflammation has spread to the periodontal ligament.
- A widened periodontal ligament may be seen on the radiographs in the later stages.

Once pulpal inflammation has spread to the periodontal ligament, the resulting inflammatory exudate may cause extrusion of the tooth, making it tender to bite on. This particular symptom, acute apical periodontitis, may be a consequence of occlusal trauma; the occlusion must therefore always be checked

Histopathology

- Acute and chronic inflammatory changes present
- Continuous vasodilatation, accompanied by the accumulation of edema fluid in the connective tissue surrounding the tiny tissue.
- Large number of WBC collection may be found beneath the area of carious penetration. Odontoblasts in this area are destroyed.

- Localized destruction of the pulp by polymorphonuclear leucocyte cells and formation of microabscess known as pulp abscess containing pus arising from the breakdown of leucocytes and bacteria as well as from digestion of tissue.

If the carious process continues to advance and penetrate the pulp, the histologic picture changes.

  - The area of ulceration is seen (chronic ulcerative pulpitis) that drains through the cavity and reduces the intrapulpal pressure and thereby the pain.
  - The liberation of proteases by lysosomes results in the formation of a pulp abscess. Changes in odontoblastic layer vary from disruption to total destruction.
  - Irreversible pulpitis progresses to necrosis.

Diagnosis

- **Pain**
  - Severity of clinical symptoms of acute pulpalgia vary as inflammatory response increases pain.
  - Mild to severe or even excruciating throbbing.
  - Continuous or has periods of cessation (intermittent).
  - Spontaneous because of the presence of necrotic tissue, which further provokes and serves as a nidus for inflammation and resultant "Suprathreshold" intrapulpal pressure increase. Thus, unlike pain of reversible pulpitis, this pain lingers after the primary (external) irritant has been removed.
  - Painful pulpitis is generally diffuse and readily not localized by the patient.
  - Patient may not be able to pinpoint the specific tooth until certain diagnostic tests are employed.

- Lying down or bending over may intensify the pain of acute pulpalgia because of overall increase in cephalic blood pressure is relayed to confined pulp tissue.
- Pain referral – painful pulpitis may be referred to other areas of the same and opposing arches as well as to structure remote from involved tooth.
- Visual examination and history may reveal previous symptoms or a traumatic experience.
- Radiographic examination: may not show anything of significance that is not already known clinically. It may disclose an interproximal cavity or caries under a filling threatening the integrity of the pulp.
- Percussion: tenderness implies an increased intrapulpal pressure, as a result of hyperactive exudative (acute) inflammatory tissue. The term acute pulpits with acute apical periodontitis are applicable in this situation.

Widening of the periodontal ligament space without percussion tenderness implies a non-painful state and the term acute pulpitis with chronic periodontitis may be used.

VITALITY TEST

Thermal test

- Irreversible pulpitis may respond in the same manner to thermal stimulation as reversible pulpitis, but pain may persist after the stimulus is removed.
- As pulpal inflammation progresses, heat will intensify the responses because it has an expansive effect on the blood vessels, tissue and gaseous products of proteolysis.

- Conversely, cold will tend to relieve the pain in advanced stages of pulpits, because, it has a contractile effect on the remaining central or apical functional vascular bed, reducing the intrapulpal pressure [9].

Electric test

- A response to less current may be expected in early stages because of low threshold of peripheral Aδ-fibres.
- As the tissue becomes more necrotic, more current is required.
- This test may not be diagnostic in advanced cases of acute pulpalgia, because of erratic mixed responses, particularly multirooted teeth.

Treatment

- Complete removal of the pulp or pulpectomy and the placement of an intracanal medicament to act as a disinfectant or obtundent.
- Surgical removal should be considered if the tooth is unrestorable.

Prognosis

Favorable if the pulp is removed and the tooth undergoes proper endodontic therapy and restoration

C. HOT TOOTH

The term "Hot tooth" is generally used for patients who are having a very painful tooth and upon treatment is persistently stubborn to fully anesthetize. In some cases, despite the area being profoundly "numb", on commencement of root canal treatment some residual sensation is still present.[4]

Clinically in this situation after the isolation of concerned tooth and following the onset access preparation patient feels nothing when the bur is in enamel. Once the bur enters dentin or possibly not until the pulp is exposed, the patient feels sharp pain. This can be very distressing for patients and they may lose faith in Dentist and treatment protocols. Also, if such a situation occurs in children, they may develop a constant fear for dental treatment for life long. While on the other hand, Dentist has to face frustration for an unsatisfactory treatment and uncooperative patient.[4]

Diagnosis: Irreversible pulpitis (symptomatic or asymptomatic)

- Teeth most difficult to anesthetize: Mandibular molars > Mandibular and maxillary premolars > Maxillary molars > Mandibular and maxillary anteriors.
- Pulpal tissue has a very concentrated sensory nerve supply, particularly in chamber.
- So, it becomes a challenge to anaesthetize a tooth with irreversible pulpitis.

Theories of Hot Tooth[4,12,37]

1. **Location:** If the area where the anesthetic is to be administered is off the target, this can lead to partial numbness or an ineffective injection.
2. **Local tissue changes because of inflammation**: Area of inflammation around the inflamed tooth causes the anesthetic to be less effective. The lowered pH of inflamed tissue reduces the amount of base form of the anesthetic available to penetrate the nerve membrane. Consequently, there is less of the ionized form within the nerve to achieve anesthesia. It can be true only in cases of swelling. This theory does have a limitation, as it does not explain injections that are distant area from the area of inflammation, also, it is unable to explain that why it is difficult to anesthetize a tooth with pulpitis with an inferior alveolar nerve block.

3. **Hyperalgesia**: This theory states that the inflammation within the tooth has altered the actual nerve making it more difficult to numb. The nerve arising in an inflamed tissue have altered resting potentials and decreased excitability thresholds. These changes are not restricted to the inflamed pulp itself but affect the entire neuronal membrane extending up to central nervous system. Local anesthetics are not sufficient to prevent impulse transmission, owing to the lowered excitability thresholds.
4. **The nervous patient**: In some cases being nervous, apprehensive or jumpy has the vicious cycle of lowering the pain threshold. Initial apprehension leads to decreased pain threshold causing anesthesia difficulties, which leads to increased apprehension, which results in loss of control and so on.
5. **Time:** In some cases it may just be a time factor, as some patients take more time than others for anesthetic to diffuse and block the sensory nerves.
6. The anesthetic solution may not penetrate to the sensory nerves that innervate the pulp, especially in mandible.
7. **The Central Core theory:** It states that nerves on the outside of the nerve bundle supply molar teeth whereas nerves on the inside supply anterior teeth. The anesthetic solution may not diffuse into the nerve trunk to reach all nerves to produce an adequate block, even if deposited at the correct site. This theory may explain the higher experimental failure rates in anterior teeth with the inferior alveolar nerve block.
8. **TTX-Resistant Channels**: Scientists have shown that there is a special class of Sodium channels on C fibers, known as tetrodotoxin-resistant (TTXr). In case of inflammation, neuroinflammatory reactions start and Sodium channel expression on C fibers shifts from TTX sensitive to TTX

resistant creating inflammatory hyperalgesia. One of the clinically significant characteristics of these Na+ channels are relatively resistant to lignocaine. After a nerve block, a patient may describe profound anesthesia of soft tissue where no inflammation is witnessed. However, entering the vital pulp chamber may initiate pain.

In "hot tooth" (irreversible pulpitis), progressive inflammation due to advancing caries leads to acute exacerbation characterized by neutrophil infiltration and release of inflammatory mediators (prostaglandins, interleukins) and neuropeptides (substance P, bradykinin, CGRP). These sensitize pulpal nociceptors, heightening pain and neuronal excitability. Assessing adequate anesthesia in such cases is challenging—though lip numbness, gingival probing, or initiating treatment are commonly used to confirm inferior alveolar nerve block (IANB), these methods are unreliable indicators of true pulpal anesthesia.[38]

However, these techniques are not very effective in determining if pulpal anesthesia has been achieved. In teeth diagnosed with a hot irreversible pulpitis, a failure to respond to the stimulus may not necessarily guarantee pulpal anesthesia. The patient may still report pain during treatment. Teeth with necrotic pulp chambers but whose root canals contain vital tissue may not be tested using the above means. In these cases, testing for pulpal anesthesia of the neighboring teeth may give the clinician an indication of the anesthetic status of the tooth to be treated.[38]

Management of Hot Tooth [37]

1. **Patient's education:** Patient should be groomed and acknowledged about the treatment so that he is mentally aware of procedures and the fear of unknown is eliminated thus reducing anxiety.

2. **Management of anxious patient:**
   a. Give short morning appointments followed by good morning breakfast.
   b. Premedication with lorazepam 1 mg (after checking interaction with other drugs) night before sleep followed by 90 minutes prior to procedure.
   c. No driving & need to be accompanied with friend/relative/escort.
   d. Extremely short or no waiting time in waiting area.
   e. Duration, only as much as patient can tolerate making sure patient feels he/she is in command.
   f. Iatrosedation: Vocal sedation- Use of sentences like "I will be careful", Talk to them as you go through procedure, avoid use of words like hurt, sharp etc., Music, Aroma, Hypnosis, Acupuncture, Relaxation techniques (deep breathing, guided imagery, progressive relaxation) will be helpful.
3. **Role of premedication:** If required anti-inflammatory can be prescribed to be taken as 1 hour before the treatment. Providing enough time between anesthetic delivery and start of procedure.
4. Before starting access preparation, a small **test cavity** can be made to ensure effectiveness of anesthesia.
5. Additional anesthetic or **supplemental injections** are necessary to achieve profound anesthesia.

Anesthesia - Hot Tooth Management[38]

Mandibular teeth present the greatest challenge in achieving effective local anesthesia. Successful pulpal anesthesia depends on the accurate delivery of the inferior alveolar nerve block (IANB), typically confirmed by soft tissue and lip numbness. Missed blocks occurring in about 5% of cases should prompt immediate reinjection before initiating treatment.

Anesthetic success for mandibular anesthesia is defined as achieving two consecutive EPT readings of 80 within 15 minutes and maintaining them for at least 60 minutes. Clinically, this means treatment can begin within 15 minutes of administering the IANB, with pulpal anesthesia lasting approximately one hour—an optimal duration for both endodontic and restorative procedures.

However, evidence indicates that even with successful IANB (lip numbness achieved) using 2% lidocaine with 1:100,000 epinephrine, anesthetic success rates remain variable approximately 53% for mandibular first molars, 61% for first premolars, and only 35% for lateral incisors.

Strategy

- Either change the local anaesthetic or change the injection technique in attempting to block the inferior alveolar nerve.
- The Gow-Gates technique has been reported to have a higher success rate than the conventional IANB, but controlled clinical studies have failed to prove its superiority.
- The Vazirani-Akinosi technique (closed mouth) also has not been shown to be superior to the conventional IANB technique. Therefore, replacing the conventional IANB injection with these techniques will not improve success in attaining pulpal anesthesia in mandibular teeth.
- Increasing the volume of the local anesthetic delivered during the IANB has also been found not to increase the incidence of pulpal anesthesia.
- Increasing the concentration of epinephrine (1:50,000), with the hopes of keeping the anesthetic agent at the injection site longer, also showed no advantage in the IANB.

Supplemental Injections[38]

When the traditional IANB fails—especially in patients with "hot teeth"—clinicians should employ supplemental anesthesia techniques to achieve adequate pulpal anesthesia. These methods are most effective when used after confirming a clinically successful IANB (evidenced by lip numbness).

A. **Intraligamentary (Periodontal Ligament)** Injection Bangerter and colleagues reported that the periodontal ligament (PDL) supplemental injection is still one of the most widely taught and used supplemental techniques. In patients with irreversible pulpitis, Cohen and colleagues reported that the supplemental PDL injections were successful 74% of the time, whereas reinjection boosted success to 96%.[12] The key to giving a successful PDL injection remains the attainment of back-pressure during the injection. Failure to get back-pressure will most likely lead to failure PDL injections are usually given using either a standard dental anesthetic syringe or a high-pressure syringe. The development of computer-controlled anesthetic delivery systems (the Wand or the Single Tooth Anesthesia [Milestone Scientific, Livingston, NJ, USA] devices) has been found to be able to deliver a PDL injection.

B. **Infiltration:** It has shown significant increase in duration of pulpal anesthesia. Other Supplemental intraligamentary or intraosseous injections are most helpful to ensure profound local anesthesia. The Intraosseous technique allows analgesic solution to be deposited directly into the cancellous bone around the apices of the tooth. It has a rapid onset and has shown extremely favorable results when used as a supplemental analgesic for the hot tooth.

Special kits have been developed that facilitate drilling a small hole through the mucosa and cortical plate to allow injection of the anesthetic solution into the cancellous bone. X-Tips consist of a drill to perforate the cortical plate combined with a guide sleeve. When the drill is withdrawn the guide sleeve is left in situ.

C. **Intrapulpal:** Major drawback of the intrapulpal injection is the need for needle to be inserted into a very sensitive and inflamed pulp. The action can, therefore, be painful. Additionally, the pulp has to be exposed to give the injection and analgesic problems may have occurred prior to this being achieved. The injection has to be given under strong backpressure. In very few cases anatomic limitations may be noticed which should be managed accordingly like dense bone or accessory innervation (mylohyoid nerve branch) Importantly, bupivacaine was found to be more potent than lidocaine in blocking TTXr channels and may be the anesthetic of choice when treating the "hot tooth".

D. **Cryotherapy**: Applying cold to the tissues lowers the temperature, causing blood vessels to contract. Cryotherapy has an additive impact of delaying brain impulses by lowering the release of chemical mediators involved in pain transmission. By reducing the activation threshold of nociceptors and the conduction velocity of pain signals, cryotherapy also produces a local anesthetic effect.

Preemptive Strategies to Improve Success of the IANB Injection[39]

Nonsteroidal Anti-inflammatory drugs (NSAIDs): Premedication with NSAIDs inhibits the cyclooxygenase enzyme, lowering prostaglandin (PG) levels, especially PGE2.

Ibuprofen: Ibuprofen, a nonselective COX inhibitor, is the safest conventional NSAID.

Ibuprofen and Acetaminophen: Acetaminophen is a popular analgesic used to control endodontic pain, increasing pain threshold through brain interaction with cannabinoid and serotoninergic pathways. Combining ibuprofen and acetaminophen is proposed as an alternative, especially for NSAIDS-sensitive individuals with gastrointestinal ulcers or hypertension.

Lornoxicam and diclofenac, both NSAIDs, have analgesic activity through cyclo-oxygenase inhibition. Preoperative administration of 8 mg LNX significantly improved the efficacy of IANBs in patients with irreversible pulpitis.

Selective Cox-2 Inhibitors: Rofecoxib and meloxicam are highly specific COX-2 inhibitors more effective than ibuprofen in reducing post-endodontic pain. Its longer analgesic efficacy, longer duration of action, lesser gastrointestinal toxicity, and lack of inhibition of platelet function and aggregation make it a preferred choice over other analgesics. About 50 mg rofecoxib was found to be more helpful in managing post-endodontic pain after 12 and 24 hours. Meloxicam has a more favorable cardiovascular safety profile in comparison to other COX-2 inhibitors.

Pretreatment with Corticosteroids: Pretreatment with Prednisolone Prednisolone, a steroidal anti-inflammatory drug, reduces inflammation by inhibiting proinflammatory cytokines and phospholipase A2 release lowering the levels of PG's and leukotriene.

Ibuprofen and Dexamethasone: Dexamethasone is a steroidal anti-inflammatory drug that blocks the COX and lipoxygenase pathway essential for PG and leukotriene synthesis.

Premedication with Nitrous Oxide and Ketamine: Nitrous oxide, a commonly used inhalation anesthetic, acts on opiate and NMDA receptors for analgesia. Ketamine, a derivative of phencyclidine, causes dissociative anesthesia by affecting nerve membranes and interacting with opioid, monoaminergic, muscarinic, and calcium channels, enhancing the anesthetic effect.

Benzodiazepines (BZDP): Benzodiazepines, like alprazolam, are used to alleviate discomfort and enhance the effectiveness of IANB by binding to specific GABA receptor sites, thereby reducing aberrant brain activity.

Acupuncture in Success of IANB: Acupuncture is a nonpharmacologic treatment used to improve the efficacy of an IANB in teeth with irreversible pulpitis and control pain in dentistry. Acupuncture involves inserting tiny needles into acupuncture sites (also called acupoints) on the body's surface. LI4 Hegu is a single acupuncture point that has long been used to relieve oral and masticatory muscle discomfort. When the needle is inserted into an acupuncture point, the patient will experience De qi (Composite of sensations felt at the needling site after adequate needle insertion with or without proper manipulation) which manifests as numbness, heaviness, or distention around the insertion site.

5.3 SYMPTOMATIC APICAL PERIODONTITIS

(Synonyms: Acute abscess, acute apical abscess, acute dentoalveolar abscess, acute periapical abscess, acute radicular abscess)

Apical periodontitis is an inflammatory disease affecting the tissues surrounding the root end of a tooth and is caused by root canal (endodontic) infection. The disease can manifest itself in different clinical ways, including the development of an acute abscess.

Recent studies in the fields of molecular and cellular microbiology and immunology have provided information to implicate a multitude of factors in the pathogenesis of symptomatic apical periodontitis, including its most severe form, the acute apical abscess. [40]

Definition

Localized collection of pus in the alveolar bone at root apex of tooth following death of pulp, with extension of infection through apical foramen in to periradicular tissue.

The Disease Process

- An abscess consists of a collection of pus into a cavity formed by tissue liquefaction.
- The terms dental abscess, dentoalveolar abscess, and odontogenic abscess are often used synonymously to describe abscesses formed in the tissues around the tooth.
- The cause may be an endodontic infection (acute apical abscess) or a periodontal infection (periodontal abscess and pericoronitis).
- Endodontic infection develops only in root canals of teeth devoid of a vital pulp due to necrosis of the dental pulp because of caries or trauma to the tooth or to removal of the pulp tissue for previous root canal treatment. Once the infection is established

in the root canal, bacteria may contact the periradicular tissues via apical and lateral foramina or root perforations and induce a chronic or acute inflammatory response.[41]

- The chronic response is usually asymptomatic and almost invariably leads to bone resorption around the root apex, which is the typical radiographic feature of apical periodontitis.
- Acute periradicular inflammation in turn usually gives rise to signs and symptoms, including pain and swelling. The acute (symptomatic) process may develop without previous chronic inflammation or may be the result of exacerbation of a previously chronic asymptomatic lesion.
- The acute abscess can be regarded as an advanced stage of the symptomatic form of apical periodontitis.
- In acute endodontic infections, not only are the involved bacteria located in the root canal, but they invade the periradicular tissues and have the potential to spread to other anatomical spaces of head and neck to form a cellulitis or phlegmon, which is a disseminating diffuse inflammatory process with pus formation.
- The purulent exudate formed in response to root canal infection spreads through the medullary bone to perforate the cortical bone and discharge into the submucous or subcutaneous soft tissue.
- In many cases, swelling develops only intraorally.
    - Maxilla → rain through buccal or palatal bone, occasionally into the maxillary sinus or the nasal cavity.
    - Mandible → Drain through buccal or lingual bone into oral cavity. However, the infectious process may also extend into fascial spaces of the head and neck and result in cellulitis and systemic signs and symptoms, with consequent complications.

Etiology[12]

- Bacterial invasion of dead pulp tissue.
- Trauma, chemical or mechanical irritation.
- Since pulp is enclosed, chamber drainage is not possible and infection continues to extend through least resistant path i.e. Apical foramen and thereby involving periodontal ligament and periradicular bone.

Symptoms

- First symptom is tenderness that can be relieved by continued slight pressure on the extruded tooth to push it back to alveolus → severe throbbing pain with small swelling on the soft tissue overlying.
- As infections proceed swellings become more pronounced beyond original site.
- If untreated infection may progress to osteitis, periostitis, cellulitis and osteomyelitis.
- The contained pus may break through to form sinus tract to open to labial or buccal mucosa.
- Swelling is usually seen in the adjacent tissue close to affected tooth, when it became extensive the resultant cellulitis occurs.
    - Maxillary anteriors → swelling of upper lip may extend to both eyelids.
    - Maxillary posteriors → check may swell to immense size distorting facial features.
    - Mandibular posteriors → Border of jaw into submaxillary region tissue and the surface of swelling become taunt or inflamed pus starts to form beneath.

- Continued liquefaction causes pressure of underlying pus and finally causes rupture
    - A gutta-percha is placed on the sinus tract and assessed radiographically which points to involved tooth.
    - Usually, confined pus takes path of least resistance in upper jaw.

Diagnosis

- From clinical examination and subjective history.
- In early stage it is difficult to locate tooth.
- Once infection is progressed to the process of periodontitis, a radiographic evaluation shows thickening of periodontal ligament space evidence of breakdown of bone or region of root apex.
- Diagnosis is made by electric test.
- Pulp testing of affected pulp is necrotic and does not respond to electric pulp testing or application of cold.
- Tooth is tender on percussion, apical mucosa is tender palpation, and tooth may be mobile and extruded.

Complications Stemming from Acute Apical Abscesses

- Acute dental abscesses have been reported to cause severe complications and even mortality.
- Mortality is more likely a result of sepsis or airway obstruction, but death due to a spreading infection leading to massive hemorrhage from the subclavian vein into the pleural cavity has been reported.
- The spread of bacteria from endodontic abscesses to other tissues may give rise to fascial plane infections.
- The most commonly affected fascial spaces are the sublingual, submandibular, buccal and pterygomandibular spaces, but

others such as the temporal, masseteric, lateral pharyngeal, and retropharyngeal spaces can be occasionally involved.

- The spread of infections of endodontic origin into the fascial spaces of the head and neck is determined by the location of the root end of the involved tooth in relation to its overlying buccal or lingual cortical plate, the thickness of the overlying bone, and the relationship of the apex to the attachment of a muscle. For example, if a mandibular molar is affected and its root apices lie closer to the lingual cortical plate and above the attachment of the mylohyoid muscle, the purulent exudate can break through the lingual cortical plate into the sublingual space. If the root apices instead lie below the attachment of the mylohyoid muscle, the infection can spread into the submandibular space. If infection affects the sublingual and submandibular spaces bilaterally as well as the submental space, a condition known as Ludwig's angina.
- Another example of abscess complications involves infections of the midface, which can be very dangerous and result in **cavernous sinus thrombosis**. This is also a life-threatening infection, in which a thrombus formed in the cavernous sinus breaks free and leads to spread of the infection.
- Other reported complications of **disseminating dental infections** include brain abscess septicemia in a patient with multiple myeloma, deep neck infection mediastinitis necrotizing fasciitis, orbital abscess and cervical spondylodiscitis with spinal epidural abscess.
- It has been suggested that some host-related factors may contribute toward increased morbidity and mortality associated with acute dental abscesses, including diabetes, chronic alcohol and tobacco consumption, malnourishment, and the use of illicit substances.

Differential Diagnosis

Periodontal Abscess and Irreversible Pulpitis

- Periodontal abscess is accumulation of pus along root surface of tooth that originates from infection in supporting structure of tooth.
- Associated with periodontal pocket and manifest by slight pain or pressure pus may exudate through the sulcus.
- Swelling is present opposite to midsection of root and gingival border.

Prognosis

Favorable, depends on degree of local involvement and tissue destruction. Pain can be relieved with adequate drainage. Tooth can be saved by endodontic treatment. In severe case combined periodontal and endodontic treatment is done.

Microbial Diversity in Acute Apical Abscesses

Culture and molecular microbiology studies have clearly demonstrated that the apical abscess microbiota is mixed and conspicuously dominated by **anaerobic bacteria** provides a compilation of the main microbiological findings from most of these studies. It is noteworthy that while some bacterial species or groups are reported in many studies, the most prevalent species vary from study to study.

At a broader taxonomic level, the large majority of the frequently detected bacterial species belong to seven different bacterial phyla, namely, the Firmicutes (e.g., genera Streptococcus, Dialister,Filifactor, and Pseudoramibacter), Bacteroidetes (e.g., genera Porphyromonas, Prevotella, and Tannerella), Fusobacteria (e.g., genera Fusobacterium and Leptotrichia),

Actinobacteria (e.g.,genera Actinomyces and Propionibacterium), Spirochaetes (e.g., genus Treponema), Synergistetes (e.g., genus Pyramidobacter and some as-yet-uncultivated phylotypes), and Proteobacteria (e.g.,genera Campylobacter and Eikenella).[41]

Histopathology

Marked infiltration of PMNL and rapid accumulation of inflammatory exudate in response to active infection. Also, some mononuclear cells are found, the chief inflammatory cells are PMNL. As more PMNL cells die pus is formed root canal is devoid of tissue and clumps of microorganisms are seen. [42]

Treatment

Treatment of acute apical abscesses involves incision for drainage and root canal treatment or extraction of the involved tooth to remove the source of infection. In some cases, drainage can be obtained through the root canal, but when swelling is present, incision for drainage should also be performed whenever possible, since this approach has been shown to produce a quicker improvement than drainage only by opening of the root canal.

- Adjunctive systemic antibiotics are not necessary in most cases of localized and uncomplicated apical abscesses; Analgesics may be prescribed for pain control.
- The selective occasions when antibiotics are indicated in cases of acute apical abscesses include the following: abscesses associated with systemic involvement, including fever, malaise, and lymphadenopathy; disseminating infections resulting in cellulitis, progressive diffuse swelling, and/or trismus; and abscesses in medically compromised patients who are at increased risk of a secondary (focal) infection following bacteremia.

- The selective occasions when antibiotics are indicated in cases of acute apical abscesses include the following: abscesses associated with systemic involvement, including fever, malaise, and lymphadenopathy; disseminating infections resulting in cellulitis progressive diffuse swelling, and/or trismus; and abscesses in medically compromised patients who are at increased risk of a secondary (focal) infection following bacteremia.
- The selection of antibiotics in clinical practice is either empirical or based on the results of microbial susceptibility testing. For diseases with known microbial causes for which the probable microbiota has been established in the literature, empirical therapy may be used. Therefore, it is preferable to opt for an antimicrobial agent whose spectrum of action includes the most detected bacteria.
- Most of the bacterial species involved with endodontic infections, including abscesses, are susceptible to penicillin. This makes these drugs the first choice for treatment of endodontic infections when allergy of the patient to penicillin has been ruled out.
- In addition, **amoxicillin** may provide more rapid improvement in pain or swelling, and patient compliance with the prescribed regimen may be better because of the longer dosage interval of amoxicillin. In even more serious cases, including life-threatening conditions, association of amoxicillin with either clavulanic acid or metronidazole may be required to achieve optimum antimicrobial effects as a result of the spectrum of action being extended to include penicillin-resistant strains.

5.4 ACUTE EXACERBATION OF CHRONIC APICAL PERIODONTITIS (PHOENIX ABSCESS)

A Phoenix abscess is an acute suppurative inflammatory condition associated with a pre-existing chronic periapical lesion, such as a granuloma or radicular cyst. Clinically, it presents as a sudden onset of severe pain, tenderness, and swelling in a tooth that may have remained asymptomatic for months or even years despite radiographic evidence of chronic apical pathology.

The term "Phoenix abscess" was first popularized by Grossman to describe the "rebirth" of acute symptoms from a previously chronic lesion.[9] This condition exemplifies the dynamic interplay between root canal infection, host defense, and iatrogenic influences, where a stable chronic lesion can suddenly destabilize into acute suppuration.[4]

Historical Perspective

- **Kakehashi et al. (1965):** Demonstrated in germ-free and conventional rats that microorganisms are essential for the development of pulpal and periapical disease, proving the microbial basis of endodontic pathology.[43]
- **Grossman (1940s–1980s):** Popularized the term "Phoenix abscess" and emphasized its clinical importance in endodontic diagnosis and treatment planning.[9]
- **Seltzer & Naidorf (1985):** Analyzed endodontic flare-ups in depth, attributing Phoenix abscess to microbial-host interactions, iatrogenic insults, and treatment-induced alterations.[44]
- **Siqueira (2003):** Described the microbial causes of flare-ups, particularly shifts in root canal flora and the role of virulent anaerobes in transforming a quiescent lesion into an acute abscess.[45]

Etiology

1. Microbial Factors[45]

- Chronic lesions usually contain Gram-positive facultatives like Enterococcus faecalis. When ecological conditions favor anaerobes (Prevotella, Porphyromonas, Fusobacterium), these rapidly growing species release endotoxins and cytotoxic metabolites, intensifying inflammation.
- Reinfection via coronal leakage or procedural contamination introduces new pathogens.
- Microbial toxins (LPS, peptidoglycan) diffuse into periapical tissues, stimulating strong inflammatory responses.

2. Host Factors[9]

- Sudden reduction in host defenses (stress, systemic illness) may precipitate flare-ups.
- Hyperactive immune response → excessive neutrophil infiltration and tissue destruction.
- Elevated RANKL/OPG ratio → enhanced osteoclastic activity and rapid bone resorption.

3. Latrogenic/Mechanical Factors[9]

- Over-instrumentation and extrusion of debris provoke acute inflammation.
- Incomplete debridement leaves necrotic material behind, maintaining irritant potential.
- Chemical accidents, such as extrusion of sodium hypochlorite beyond the apex, can aggravate periapical tissues.

Pathogenesis

1. Microbial Equilibrium and Disturbance[45]

Following pulp necrosis, microorganisms colonize the root canal system. Their antigens diffuse through the apex, establishing chronic granulomatous inflammation. When equilibrium is disrupted—by microbial shifts, reinfection, or mechanical irritation—the lesion flares up into acute suppuration.

2. Host Immune Response[9,45]

- **Antigen recognition:** Pattern recognition receptors (PRRs) detect microbial molecules, activating NF-κB and promoting cytokine production.
- **Neutrophil response:** Large neutrophil influx leads to ROS and protease release, killing microbes but also damaging host tissue, causing liquefaction necrosis and pus.
- **Vascular changes:** Histamine, bradykinin, and prostaglandins increase permeability, producing edema, pressure, and severe throbbing pain.

3. Bone Destruction[9]

- Cytokines and prostaglandins induce osteoblasts and stromal cells to express RANKL, activating osteoclasts. The raised RANKL/OPG ratio accelerates bone resorption.
- Matrix metalloproteinases (MMPs) from neutrophils further degrade collagen in the periodontal ligament and bone.

Symptoms[9]

- **Pain:** Severe, throbbing, continuous; aggravated by chewing, percussion, or lying down. Radiates to the jaw, temple, or ear.
- **Tenderness/pressure:** Patients describe the tooth as "raised" due to periapical edema.[85]

- **Swelling:** Initially localized; may progress intraorally or extraorally with pus accumulation.
- **Systemic signs:** Fever, malaise, lymphadenopathy, or trismus in severe cases.

Signs[9]

- **Tooth vitality:** The affected tooth is non-vital and acutely tender to percussion and palpation.
- **Mobility:** Mild mobility due to widened periodontal ligament space.
- **Radiographs:** Pre-existing lesion visible; acute exacerbation shows widened PDL space, loss of sharp radiolucency borders.
- **Suppuration:** Fluctuant swelling indicates pus; sinus tract may form later if drainage occurs.

Differential Diagnosis[9]

- **Phoenix abscess vs Acute apical abscess:** Phoenix arises from a pre-existing chronic lesion; acute apical abscess can develop in a recently necrotic tooth without prior radiographic changes.
- **Phoenix abscess vs Periodontal abscess:** The latter shows periodontal pocketing with a vital pulp, distinguishing it from Phoenix abscess.

Management of Phoenix Abscess[9]

The management of Phoenix abscess aims to:

1. **Relieve pain and swelling**
2. **Eliminate infection**
3. **Establish drainage**
4. **Preserve the tooth whenever possible**

1. Emergency Management

- **Establish Drainage**
  - The most important step is to relieve intraosseous pressure by allowing pus to escape.
  - Drainage can be achieved through the root canal system after gaining access to the pulp chamber.
  - If drainage through the canal is incomplete, an **incision and drainage (I&D)** procedure is indicated to evacuate pus from the soft tissues.
- **Trephination (rarely used)** may be considered in severe localized swellings not relieved by canal or incision drainage.

2. Root Canal Therapy

- **Cleaning and shaping:** Thorough debridement of the canal system removes necrotic tissue and microbial irritants.
- **Irrigation:** Copious irrigation with sodium hypochlorite is essential to flush out debris and disinfect the canal.
- **Intracanal medicament:** Placement of calcium hydroxide between appointments provides antibacterial action and reduces inflammation.
- **Obturation:** Should be postponed until the infection subsides and the canal is dry and asymptomatic.

3. Pharmacologic Support

- **Analgesics:** NSAIDs are effective for pain control by reducing prostaglandin-mediated inflammation.
- **Antibiotics:** Generally not required if effective drainage is established.

- Indicated only in cases of spreading infection, cellulitis, systemic involvement (fever, lymphadenopathy, malaise), or in immunocompromised patients.
- Amoxicillin (or clindamycin in penicillin-allergic patients) is commonly prescribed when indicated.

4. Adjunctive Measures

- Warm saline rinses may promote drainage and patient comfort.
- Occlusal adjustment can help reduce pain from traumatic occlusion caused by extrusion of the tooth.
- Follow-up is essential to confirm healing and prevent recurrence.

5. Surgical Options

- If root canal therapy fails or if the lesion persists despite treatment, **periapical surgery** (apicoectomy with retrograde filling) may be required to remove persistent periapical infection.

Prognosis[45]

- With proper drainage and endodontic therapy, prognosis is excellent, and the lesion usually heals completely.
- Delayed or inadequate treatment may allow the infection to spread, causing cellulitis, osteomyelitis, or systemic complications.

5.5 CRACKED TOOTH SYNDROME

Cracked tooth is defined as an incomplete fracture of the dentine in a vital posterior tooth that involves the dentine and occasionally extends into the pulp. The term "cracked tooth syndrome" (CTS) was first introduced by Cameron in 1964. The diagnosis of CTS is often problematic and has been known to challenge even the most experienced dental operators, accountable largely by the fact that the associated symptoms tend to be very variable and at times bizarre.[46]

Etiology. -Several factors facilitate the development of CTS.[46]

Table 5.1

CLASSIFICATION	FACTORS	EXAMPLES
Restorative Procedures	Inadequate design features	1. Over-preparation of cavities 2. Deep cusp fossa relationship 3. Insufficient cuspal protection in inlay/onlay design
	Stress concentration	1. Pin placement (Friction lock or self threading dentin pins) 2. Non-incremental application of composite resins 3. Pressure exerted during the seating of tightly fitting cast restorations

CLASSIFICATION	FACTORS	EXAMPLES
Occlusal Factors	A. Masticatory trauma	1. Sudden and excessive cutting force on a piece of hard object (bone)
	B. Trauma from occlusion	1. Eccentric contacts and interferences (especially mandibular second molars)
	C. Functional forces	1. Large untreated carious lesion 2. Cyclic forces
	D. Parafunctional Habit	1.Bruxism and bruxomania
Developmental factors	A. Incomplete fusion of areas of Calcification	1. Occurence of cracked tooth syndrome in unrestored tooth or teeth with minor restoration
Miscellaneous Factors	A. Thermal cycling	1. Enamel cracks
	B. Foreign body	1. Lingual barbella
	C. Dental instrument	High speed rotary instruments associated crazing and cracking

Diagnosis

- Identification can be difficult because the discomfort or pain can mimic that arising from other pathologies, such as sinusitis, temporomandibular joint disorders, headaches, ear pain, or atypical orofacial pain.
- Early diagnosis is paramount as restorative intervention can limit propagation of the fracture, subsequent microleakage and involvement of the pulpal or periodontal tissues, or catastrophic failure of the cusp.[47]
- The ease of diagnosis varies according to the position and extent of the fracture. Mandibular second molars, followed by mandibular first molars and maxillary premolars are the most commonly affected teeth.
- Early diagnosis is linked to successful restoration and a good prognosis.
- Factors contributing to an accurate diagnosis include a careful history and assessment of symptoms, especially with respect to cold sensitivity and sharp pain with forceful biting.
- Fractures tend to line up parallel to the forces on the cuspal incline. Cracks are more likely to be superficial in larger restorations, producing fewer symptoms.
- Smaller restorations tend to have deeper cracks located closer to the pulp. Vertical cracks are more common and tend to run in a mesiodistal direction along the occlusal surface, involving one or both marginal ridges.
- Among the other conditions mimicking CTS are acute periodontal disease, reversible pulpitis, dentinal hypersensitivity, galvanic pain related to silver amalgam restorations, postoperative sensitivity caused by microleakage of composite resin, fractured restorations, areas of hyper occlusion, occlusal trauma through

parafunctional tooth grinding, and orofacial pain from conditions like trigeminal neuralgia and psychiatric disorders.

The Commonly Presenting Signs and Symptoms Seen in Cases of Cracked Tooth Syndrome[48]

- Sudden, sharp pain on biting/chewing and in some cases on release: 'rebound pain'
- Sensitivity to cold thermal stimuli; in some cases, hyper-reactivity to hot/sugary stimuli may also occur
- Symptoms may be present for periods ranging from weeks to months
- Inconsistent ability to localize the affected tooth
- Pain may be elicited by lateral cusp pressure, as evoked by 'bite test' and tooth grinding
- Fracture lincs may be seen clinically (sometimes upon removal of the restoration), aided by magnification,
- dyes or transillumination
- Positive response to vitality tests; exaggerated response to cold thermal stimuli
- Radiographs; usually inconclusive

Other clues evident on examination include the presence of facets on the occlusal surfaces of teeth (identifies teeth involved in eccentric contact and at risk from damaging lateral forces), the presence of localized periodontal defects (found where cracks extend subgingivally), or the evocation of symptoms by sweet or thermal stimuli. The use of rubber dam enhances the probability of visualizing these cracks by isolating the tooth, highlighting the crack with a contrasting background, keeping the area free of saliva, and reducing peripheral distractions.

Visual Inspection[46]

Visual inspection of the tooth is useful, but cracks are not often visible without the aid of magnifying loupes, it can be occasionally detected.

Tactile Examination[46]

Scratch the surface of the tooth with the tip of a sharp explorer. The tip may catch in a crack.

a) Exploratory Excavation[46]

- Sometimes exploratory excavation becomes necessary to obtain a visual diagnosis.
- The decision to excavate should always be made with the consent of the patient since it is not guaranteed that a fracture will be found underneath any removed restoration. Removal of existing restorations may reveal fracture lines.

b) Periodontal Probing[46]

- Periodontal probing helps distinguish between a cracked tooth and a split tooth when the fracture line extends below the gingiva, thereby causing a localized periodontal defect.
- For suspected cracks, careful probing must be performed to disclose the presence of an isolated periodontal pocket.
- However, isolated deep probing often indicates the presence of split tooth, which predicts a poor prognosis.

Dye Test[46]

- Gentian Violet or methylene blue stains can be used to highlight fracture lines.
- The disadvantage of this technique is that it takes at least 2–5 days to be effective and may require placement of a provisional restoration.

- Placing a provisional restoration undermines the structural integrity of the tooth and further propagates the crack.
- An additional disadvantage is that a definitive esthetic restoration cannot be obtained.

Transillumination[46]

- Transillumination is an important aid in locating the crack whether it is incomplete, as in CTS, or a complete vertical root fracture.
- When performing transillumination, the tooth should be cleaned and the light source placed directly on the tooth.
- A crack that penetrates into the dentin of the tooth will cause a disruption in the light transmission under these circumstances.
- Transillumination is probably the most common modality for traditional crack diagnosis.

Drawbacks To Using Transillumination Without Magnification

1. Transillumination dramatizes all cracks to the point that craze lines appear as structural cracks.
2. Subtle color changes are rendered invisible. Transillumination with a fiber-optic light and use of magnification will aid in visualization of a crack.

Bite Tests[46]

- Symptom mimickers can be used to reproduce the symptoms associated with incomplete fractures of posterior teeth.
- Bite tests can be performed using orange wood sticks, cotton wool rolls, rubber abrasive wheels such as Berlew wheels, or the head of number 10 round bur in a handle of cellophane tape.
- When using orange wood sticks to determine cracks, the patient is asked to bite on individual cusps separately. This helps to

isolate the fractured cusp. Cotton rolls can be used to detect cracks.

- The patient is asked to bite down on cotton rolls and then suddenly release the pressure.
- Pain perceived on sudden release of pressure confirms the diagnosis.
- The use of rubber plungers of anesthetic carpules suspended from a length of floss can be used in a similar manner as that of cotton rolls.
- Tooth slooth can be used on each individual cusp and the patient is asked to bite, thus allowing the placement of selective pressure on one cusp.
- If there is pain on biting or release of biting pressure, it is indicative that the cusp is cracked. Vitality tests are usually positive.
- However, sometimes the affected teeth may display hypersensitivity to cold stimuli due to the presence of pulpal inflammation, a feature that may help to confirm a diagnosis of CTS.

Radiograph[46]

- Radiographs can aid in evaluating the pulpal and periodontal health of a tooth, but it is rare to see a crack on a radiograph.
- Radiographs tend to be of limited use as fractures tend to propagate in a mesiodistal direction, parallel to that of the plane of the film.
- However, they can be useful in detecting more rarely occurring fractures which may run in a buccolingual direction and for excluding other dental pathology.

Microscopic Detection[46]

- Experienced clinicians using a clinical microscope have reached a general consensus that ×16 provides an ideal magnification level for the evaluation of enamel cracks, with a range from ×14 to ×18.
- Use of the clinical microscope makes possible the treatment of asymptomatic but structurally unsound posterior teeth.
- Ultrasound is also capable of imaging cracks in simulated tooth structure and could pose an important diagnostic aid in the future.
- Where direct diagnostic methods prove unsuccessful, indirect diagnostic methods like banding can be used to detect CTS.

Differentiating a Cracked Tooth from a Fractured Cusp or Split Tooth

- If a crack can be detected, use wedging to test for movement of the segments to differentiate a cracked tooth from a fractured cusp or split tooth.
- No movement with wedging forces implies a cracked tooth.
- A fractured cusp may break off under slight pressure with no further mobility.
- A split tooth will show mobility with wedging forces and the mobile segment extends well below the cemento-enamel junction

Where removal of the fractured cusp is to be undertaken, it should be performed with extreme caution, as there is a risk of attenuation of the fracture plane. Subtractive occlusal adjustment is invasive and will not help to avoid the continual flexure of the tooth upon loading when an occlusal load is applied. Cusp reduction to overlay it with a protective restorative material may be required: composite 2 mm, gold and other alloys 1 mm

Management of CTS

Immediate Management of CTS

- Traditionally, unless the affected cusp has been splintered off during the removal of an existing restoration when undertaking exploratory procedure, acute management has generally been provided using immediate extra-coronal circumferential splints (such as copper rings, orthodontic bands or provisional crowns) or by the application of direct (intra-coronal or extra-coronal splints) usually involving some form of tooth preparation, where some biological compromise is likely to be incurred.

Direct Intra-Coronal Restorations

- When using an intra-coronal restoration to treat an incompletely fractured posterior tooth, the objective is to anchor the chosen dental material to the cavity walls at either side of the fracture plane.
- This would help to not only prevent the independent movement of the portions either side of the fracture plane, but also aid in restoring the intrinsic fracture toughness of a tooth.
- There is some evidence to support the short-term prescription of direct, resin bonded posterior composite restorations to treat cases of CTS.

The Longer-Term Management of CTS

- Placement of a restoration that provides cuspal coverage has the potential to restore the fracture toughness of a restored tooth to that of an intact tooth.
- In case of a posterior tooth with a crack that has extended into dentine, it is reasonable to assume that the fracture toughness

of the affected tooth is likely to be undermined; this may be achieved by an onlay, overlay or crown restoration.

- Restorations that provide cuspal coverage may be fabricated directly or indirectly.

A. The Use of Direct Onlay Restorations to Treat CTS

The use of direct materials to provide longer-term management of CTS has a number of clear merits.

Restorations may be placed in a single visit; this may prove time effective.
Provisional restorations are avoided; provisional restorations are not as well adapted as definitive restorations, which may facilitate the continual ingress of noxious stimuli or microorganisms into the crack. Provisional restorations will nether provide the same level of cuspal support as a definitive restoration formed from a more robust dental material.
Costly laboratory fees are averted.

Merits of Direct Onlay Restorations for the Management of CTS

- Direct onlays used to treat incompletely fractured posterior teeth may be formed using silver amalgam[30] or resin composite.[26]
- The direct composite onlay restoration therefore offers a lesser invasive and aesthetic alternative to use of dental amalgam overlays for this purpose.
- It is likely that a reduction in the height of the affected cusp will reduce the leverage placed on it when an occlusal load is applied, while its coverage with a plastic material will not only provide a form of 'shock absorption' but also help to divert occlusal loads from the crack towards the axial walls (to which the overlay will be anchored) and ultimately down the long axis of the tooth (which may in turn also lessen the stresses applied to the adhesive interface) and optimize restoration longevity.

B. Indirect Restorations with Cuspal Coverage

- Indirect techniques offer the use of dental materials which have the potential to offer superior mechanical properties in the oral environment, and are perhaps less demanding of operator skill versus the use and placement of direct onlay restorations.
- When using occlusal coverage restorations, the cusp angle should be reduced to reduce the risk of lateral loading.
- The use of ceramic onlays to treat CTS should perhaps be undertaken with an element of caution.
- Ceramics are relatively brittle materials that display limited ability of plastic deformation under load.
- Ceramics are less likely to offer desirable 'shock absorbing' properties, with the possibility of an incomplete alleviation of symptoms as well as the risks of continued fracture propagation.
- Intra-oral adjustments with dental ceramic materials may be challenging.
- Indirect composite onlays may provide an aesthetic alternative to the use of ceramic, with the merits of ease of adjustment, and repair.
- Indirect adhesive onlay techniques offer a more conservative alternative to full coverage restorations.
- The use of in-surgery CAD/CAM manufacturing techniques may however, offer some potential by overcoming difficulties such as the challenges associated with provisionalisation which may increase the risks of pulpal complications among incompletely fractured teeth.
- The prescription of full coverage crowns has been suggested to be the most suitable form of treatment for the management of CTS, owing to their potential ability of the resistance form provided by such restorations to help dissipate applied occlusal loads over the entire prepared tooth as well as the retention form (by frictional contact) to provide effectual immobilization.

C. A Novel Ultra-Conservative Approach to the Management of CTS

The clinical steps involved for this technique include.

- Confirming the complete elimination of the symptoms of rebound pain from the diagnosed tooth with a non-bonded composite splint.
- Evaluation of the periapical status and bone support with an accurate long cone periapical radiograph.
- An explanation of the technique should be provided to the patient, outlining the nature of the treatment along with instructions for anticipating the change in their occlusal scheme.
- The application of a slurry of pumice the occlusal and axial walls of the diagnosed tooth, or the alternative use of air-abrasion techniques
- Conditioning for adhesive bonding using a total etch technique, involving the use of 37% phosphoric applied over the occlusal and the axial walls for 20 seconds, followed by thoroughly washing the surfaces and the subsequent drying of the etched surfaces.
- Placement and curing of the chosen bonding resin as per the manufacturers' instructions
- Placement of a composite resin on the occlusal surface and 2–3 mm down the axial walls (buccal, palatal/lingual). The depth of composite resin placed on the occlusal surface should be to 1.0–1.5 mm in thickness, along the axial walls composite to finish in an infinity bevel and supragingivally. Light cure to manufacturers' instructions.
- The occlusal surface should to remain 'flat' with the absence of any contact during any excursive mandibular movements.

(condt.)

In certain instances, a canine rise may be added in composite to achieve this

- Composite to be polished.
- The patient should be reviewed within in one week to confirm alleviation of symptoms, followed by a periodic review every two weeks until all other tooth contacts are re-established
- Substitution of the composite splint with a definitive adhesive restoration once other tooth contacts reestablished. Remove canine rise restoration if required.

The diagnosis and management of CTS in dental practice can sometimes prove to be highly taxing on the operator. There is a need for an effective technique to provide immobilization. The DCS restoration may have considerable merits for the diagnosis and management of CTS in a predictable and minimally invasive manner.

5.6 TRAUMATIC INJURY LEADING TO CROWN AND ROOT FRACTURE

Traumatic injuries to teeth can involve several dental and peri-radicular tissues, leading to complex patterns of damage and healing. A thorough understanding of the biological responses of these tissues is essential for effective management. Dental trauma most commonly affects children between 7 and 12 years of age and is usually caused by falls or minor accidents occurring near home or school. The anterior region of the mouth, particularly the maxillary teeth, is most frequently involved. More severe incidents, such as road traffic accidents, may affect any tooth across all age groups.[49]treatment planning and followup are important for improving a favorable outcome. Guidelines should assist dentists and patients in decision making and for providing the best care effectively and efficiently. The International Association of Dental Traumatology (IADT)

Following trauma, endodontic intervention is often required in caries-free, single-rooted young permanent teeth. When prompt and appropriate care is provided, the prognosis for these teeth is generally favourable. Traumatic dental injuries are broadly classified into two main categories: fractures and luxation injuries. Fractures are further divided into crown, crown-root, and root types. Fractures involving pulp exposure are termed complicated fractures, while those without exposure are known as uncomplicated fractures.[49]treatment planning and followup are important for improving a favorable outcome. Guidelines should assist dentists and patients in decision making and for providing the best care effectively and efficiently. The International Association of Dental Traumatology (IADT)

CLASSIFICATION

1. Classification of Injuries to Anterior Teeth by Ellis and Davey[50]

Class	Description
Class I	Simple fracture of crown involving only enamel with little or no dentin
Class II	Extensive fracture of crown involving considerable dentin but not exposing dental pulp
Class III	Extensive fracture of crown involving considerable dentin and exposing dental pulp
Class IV	The traumatized tooth that becomes non vital with or without loss of crown structure
Class V	Total tooth loss – avulsion
Class IX	Traumatic injuries of primary teeth

2. Classification By Garcia- Godoy[83]

Class 0	Enamel crack
Class 1	Enamel fracture
Class 2	Enamel – dentin fracture without pulp exposure
Class 3	Enamel – dentin fracture with pulp exposure
Class 4	Enamel dentin – cementum fracture without pulp exposure
Class 5	Enamel dentin cementum fracture with pulp exposure

Class 6	Root fracture
Class 7	Concussion
Class 8	Luxation
Class 9	Lateral displacement
Class 10	Intrusion
Class 11	Extrusion
Class 12	Avulsion

3. Classification By WHO (1994)[83]

873.60	Enamel fracture
873.61	Enamel and dentin fracture without pulp exposure
873.62	Enamel and dentin fracture with pulp exposure
873.63	Root fracture
873.64	Crown-root fracture
873.66	Concussion, luxation
873.67	Intrusion, extrusion
873.68	Avulsion
873.69	Soft tissue injuries

4. Classification according to the International Classification of Diseases (1992)

Table 5.2

Type/Class	Code	Description
Enamel infraction	N 502.50	An incomplete fracture (crack) of the enamel without loss of tooth substance
Enamel fracture (uncomplicated crown fracture)	N 502.50	A fracture with loss of tooth substance confined to the enamel
Enamel–dentin fracture (uncomplicated crown fracture)	EN 502.51	A fracture with loss of tooth substance confined to enamel and dentin but not involving the pulp
Complicated crown fracture	N 502.52	A fracture involving enamel and dentin and exposing the pulp
Complicated crown–root fracture	N 502.54	A fracture involving enamel–dentin and cementum and exposing the pulp
Root fracture	N 503.53	A fracture involving dentin, cementum and the pulp
Concussion	N 503.20	An injury to the tooth-supporting structures without abnormal loosening or displacement of the tooth, but with marked reaction to percussion

Type/Class	**Code**	**Description**
Subluxation	N 503.20	An injury to the tooth-supporting structures with abnormal loosening, but without displacement of the tooth
Extrusive luxation (Peripheral dislocation, partial avulsion)	N 503.20	Partial displacement of the tooth out of its socket
Lateral luxation	N 503.20	Displacement of the tooth in a direction other than axillary, accompanied by communication or fracture of the alveolar socket
Intrusive luxation (Central dislocation)	N 503.21	Displacement of the tooth into the alveolar bone, accompanied by comminuting or fracture of the alveolar socket
Avulsion (Exarticulation)	N 503.22	Complete displacement of the tooth out of its socket
Fracture of mandibular or maxillary alveolar socket wall	N 502.40 N502.60	A fracture confined to the facial or oral socket wall

Crown Fractures

Fractures limited to the crown of a tooth (enamel ± dentin, with or without pulp exposure) most frequently affect young, caries-free anterior teeth (permanent incisors). Preservation or re-establishment of pulp vitality is a primary objective because it directly influences long-term prognosis. In cases of trauma where the pulp remains vital or is exposed yet manageable, vital pulp therapy — such as partial pulpotomy or direct pulp capping with bioactive materials — is indicated. The literature demonstrates that when correctly performed and followed-up, this approach supports favourable outcomes in such crown fractures. [51]

In practice: after fragment retrieval (if available) and stabilization, a bonded restoration or re-attachment may be undertaken; if pulp exposure is present and the root apices are open or closed, partial pulpotomy or full pulpotomy is selected appropriately, followed by definitive restoration.[52]

Crown-Root Fractures

A crown-root fracture involves the enamel, dentin and cementum, often extending below the gingival margin and involving or not involving the pulp.[53] Initial management focuses on periodontal and restorative considerations: establishing a sound, accessible margin and adequate ferrule/restoration design. If periodontally the tooth remains maintainable (i.e., healthy tissue support, manageable fracture line), then pulp management mirrors that of a pure crown fracture: vital pulp therapy if pulp is still vital, or root-canal treatment if pulp necrosis is present.[53]

Key considerations include the depth of the fracture, position relative to the alveolar crest, ability to isolate for restoration, and whether surgical or orthodontic extrusion is needed to expose sufficient tooth structure.[53]

Root Fractures

A root fracture is a horizontal (or oblique) fracture line located somewhere along the root (cervical, middle or apical third), potentially separating the coronal and apical segments.[54,55] Contrary to what might be assumed, a substantial number of pulps in root-fractured teeth will maintain vitality after such trauma. Typically the apical segment remains vital, and in many cases the coronal segment either remains vital or regains vitality over time.[54,55] Should the coronal segment lose vitality permanently (and root development is incomplete), management should follow protocols for non-vital immature permanent teeth (for example apexification or revascularisation). The apical fragment very rarely requires treatment.[54,55]

Therapeutic protocol: reposition displaced fragments promptly, apply a flexible splint (approximately 4 weeks; longer if the fracture is in cervical third), monitor pulp vitality and periapical status long-term (minimum 1-year recommended). If pulp necrosis of the coronal fragment occurs, conventional endodontic treatment to the fracture line is indicated.[54,55]

Luxation Injuries and Avulsion

Luxation injuries (extrusive, lateral, intrusive) and avulsion represent more severe dental trauma. These injuries often result in pulp necrosis and disruption of the cemental/periodontal protective layer of the root surface. The lack of this cemental/periodontal protection increases the risk of bacterial invasion and external root resorption (inflammatory or replacement types) — hence these injuries carry a potentially catastrophic prognosis if not managed correctly.[56]

Emergency management and subsequent follow-up are vital. The clinical aim is to reposition the tooth (or replanted tooth), apply an appropriate flexible splint for the indicated period (depending on displacement and root development), monitor for pulp necrosis and resorption, and initiate root-canal treatment timely when indicated (especially in mature apices).[56]

Emergency Care: Initial Evaluation Checklist[56,57]

Before proceeding for definitive treatment, a thorough evaluation must be completed, which includes:

1. Patient identifiers: name, age, sex, address, contact numbers (and weight in young/paediatric patients if sedation/anaesthesia may be required)
2. Assessment of Central nervous system : any loss of consciousness, vomiting, amnesia, dizziness following the trauma
3. General health status: systemic conditions, bleeding disorders, medications, allergies
4. Injury details: time of incident, location, mechanism of injury
5. Any prior treatment: first aid, dental care already provided elsewhere
6. History of previous dental injuries: previous fractures, luxations or restorations in the involved region
7. Occlusal/bite disturbances: new or altered occlusion, mobility or displaced segments
8. Pulp sensitivity/reaction: response to thermal testing, sweet/sour stimuli (if feasible)
9. Pain on palpation/percussion or during eating: soreness to touch or mastication
10. Spontaneous dental pain: pain without provocation indicating possible pulpal or periodontal involvement

Diagnosis of Traumatic Injury

For decades, the validity of thermal and electric tests on traumatized teeth has been under controversy. Only generalized impressions may be gained from these tests following a traumatic injury. In reality sensitivity tests for nerve function do not indicate the presence or absence of blood circulation within the pulpal space. It is assumed that after a traumatic injury, the conduction capability of the nerve endings and/or sensory receptors is usually deranged to inhibit the nerve impulse from an electric or thermal stimulus, which makes the traumatized tooth vulnerable to false negative readings. [58]

Teeth that give a response at the initial examination cannot be assumed to be healthy and continue to give a response over time similarly teeth that yield no response cannot be assumed to have necrotic pulps, because they may give a response at later follow-up visits. It has been demonstrated that it may take as long as 9 months for normal blood flow to return to the coronal pulp of a traumatized fully formed tooth. As circulation is restored, the responsiveness to pulp tests is noted. [55,59,60]

Thermal and electric pulp tests of all anterior teeth (canine to canine) of the maxillary and mandibular jaws should be performed at the time of the initial examination and carefully recorded. This serves as a baseline record which aids to compare with the results obtained in the subsequent repeated tests done at 3 weeks, at 3, 6, and 12 months, and at yearly intervals following the trauma.[58]

The purpose of these tests is to establish a trend as to the physiologic status of the pulps of these teeth. Particularly in traumatized teeth, carbon dioxide snow (CO2, -78° C) or dichlorodifluoromethane (-40° C) placed on the incisal third of the facial surface gives more accurate response.[61]

The electric pulp test relies on electric impulses directly stimulating the nerves of the pulp. These tests have limited value in young teeth but are useful in cases where the dentinal tubules are closed and do not allow dentinal fluid to flow in them. This situation is typical of teeth in elderly patients or in traumatized teeth that are undergoing premature sclerosis. In these situations, the thermal tests that rely on fluid flow in the tubules cannot be used, and the electric pulp test becomes important.[58]

Radiographs are another essential tool in the thorough examination of traumatized hard tissues. They may reveal root fractures, subgingival crown fractures, tooth displacements, bone fractures, resorptions of the root, and adjacent bone or foreign objects.[62]

According to new guidelines by, the International Association of Dental Traumatology (IADT), four different radiographs are recommended for almost every injury. AAE guidelines recommend taking one occlusal and two periapical radiographs with different lateral angulations for all dental injuries, including crown fractures. If cone beam-computed tomography is available, it should be considered for more serious injuries like crown/root, root and alveolar fractures, as well as all luxation injuries.[62]

Once the diagnosis has been established and more severe conditions—such as central nervous system involvement or fractures of the jaws and facial bones—have been excluded, the **emergency phase of management** should begin. The **primary objective** in the treatment of dental trauma is the preservation or restoration of **pulp vitality** in the affected teeth. This is particularly important because traumatic dental injuries most often occur in **children and adolescents**, whose teeth are still in the process of root development. If pulpal vitality is lost at this stage, **root maturation ceases**, potentially compromising the long-term prognosis of the tooth.[62]

Treatment

Crown Fractures

In cases of **crown or crown–root fractures**, the initial step is to **locate and preserve the fractured tooth fragment**. With the advent of **advanced adhesive and bonding techniques**, it is often possible to **reattach the fragment** to the remaining tooth structure—an approach that offers superior **esthetic and functional results**. Before reattachment, a **clinical and radiographic evaluation** should be performed to determine the **thickness of the remaining dentin** covering the pulp. When at least **0.5 mm of dentin** remains intact, placement of a protective liner is generally unnecessary. However, if the **residual dentin is less than 0.5 mm**, the deepest portion adjacent to the pulp should be covered with a **calcium hydroxide or glass ionomer liner** to provide protection. In more **complicated fractures**, it is crucial to establish a **bacteria-tight seal** after carefully cleaning the pulpal wound and removing all inflamed tissue, thereby safeguarding the **vitality of the pulp** and promoting optimal healing.[63]

Currently, the most widely accepted **pulp capping materials** are **calcium hydroxide** and **mineral trioxide aggregate (MTA)**, both of which demonstrate excellent **biocompatibility and dentin bridge formation**. In recent years, **newer bioceramic-based materials** have also shown promising results for vital pulp therapy.[64]

It is recommended to prepare a **1–2 mm deep cavity or reservoir** into the pulp chamber using a **high-speed diamond bur with copious water irrigation** to minimize heat generation. The selected capping material is then gently placed into the prepared site, after which the **tooth fragment may be reattached** or the **crown restored using composite resin**.[65]

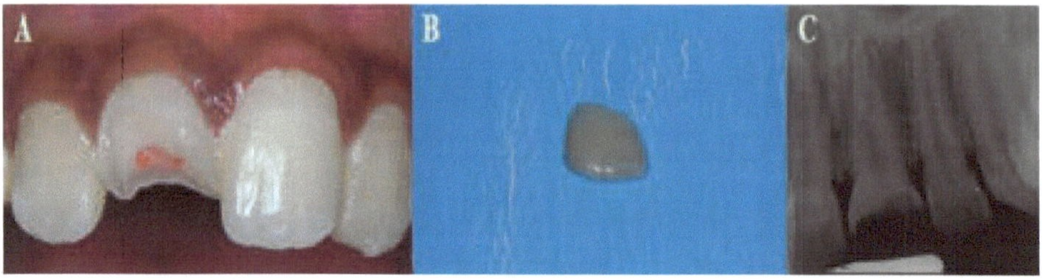

Figure 3: (A,B,C): Preoperative Photographs and radiograph

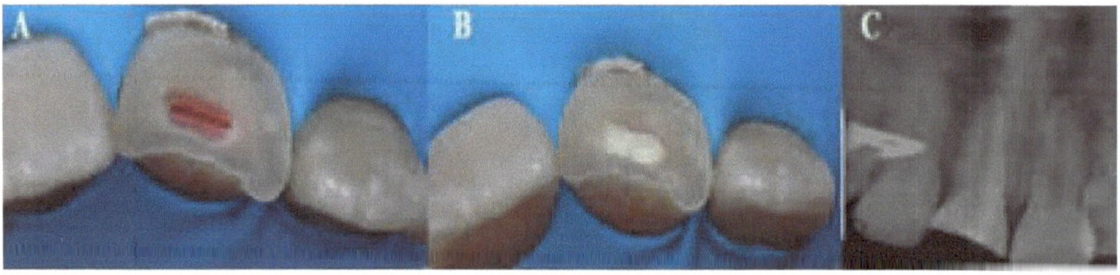

Figure 4: A) Partial Pulmotomy, B) Placement of MTA, C) Radigraph after MTA

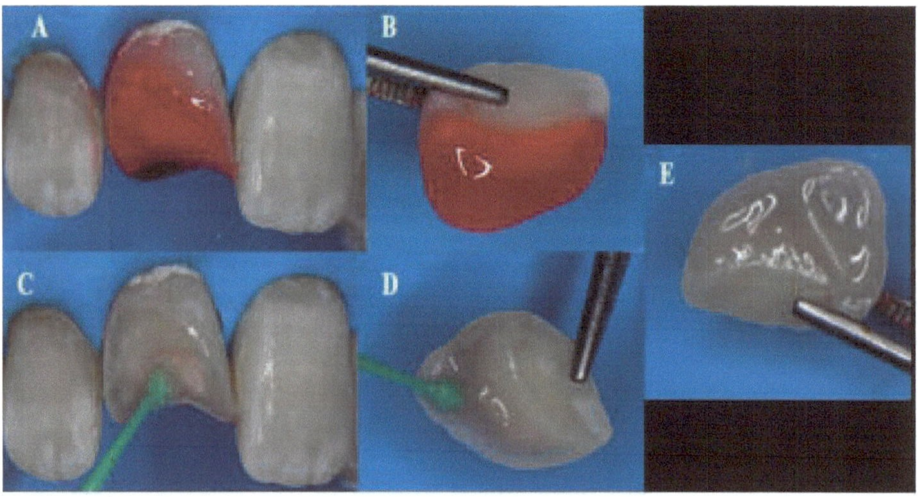

Figure 5: A,B) etching with 37% phosphoric acid, C,D) application of bonding agent, E) application of flowable composite

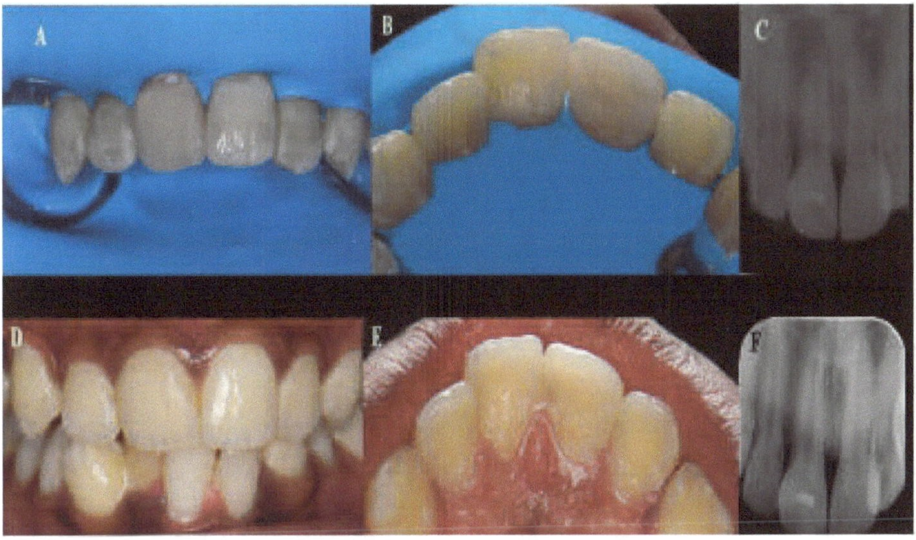

Figure 6: A,B,C) Immediate follow up, C,D,E) Follow up after 6 months Crown-Root Fractures

Crown-Root Fractures

Among the various types of dental fractures, crown–root fractures are often the most challenging to manage, primarily because the fracture margin must be exposed circumferentially around the tooth to allow for proper restoration. When the fracture line extends into the gingival sulcus, exposure can be achieved through a gingivectomy. In more extensive cases, however, orthodontic extrusion or surgical repositioning may be necessary to elevate the fracture line above the gingival margin.[62]

During the emergency phase, if the pulp is exposed, it should be protected in the same manner as in complicated crown fractures. In cases without pulpal exposure, any exposed dentin should be covered with a suitable lining material to improve patient comfort and minimize sensitivity. Generally, pulpal survival in these fracture types is favourable, although endodontic therapy may later become necessary. It is therefore essential to establish a regular recall schedule and perform pulp vitality testing at each visit to monitor healing.[62]

Root Fractures

In all root fracture cases, the pulpal tissue is affected to some extent. However, if the fractured fragments are repositioned promptly and accurately, the pulp often revascularizes across the fracture line, and endodontic intervention may not be required. Studies indicate that successful outcomes are achievable regardless of patient age, provided that proper approximation is achieved soon after injury. A retrospective clinical study evaluating the type and duration of splinting in root fractures found that when the coronal fragment remains stable after repositioning, either no splinting or a flexible splint for about two weeks yields the most favorable prognosis. Longer splinting periods are recommended only when the fracture is located near the cervical region of the tooth, where stabilization is more critical for healing.[62]

Luxation Injuries

All luxation injuries result in some degree of trauma to the periodontal ligament (PDL) and, in certain cases, to the dental pulp as well. Immediate management should aim to minimize additional damage to the PDL and promote the best possible conditions for healing. As with all traumatic dental injuries, systematic follow-up is essential, since late complications such as internal or external root resorption are relatively common and may necessitate endodontic therapy. Referral to an endodontist is recommended in complex or severe cases.[54]

Luxation injuries are categorized primarily based on severity. The mildest forms are concussion and subluxation. In both, the tooth remains in its socket but is tender to percussion; in subluxation, increased mobility is observed. No immediate treatment is generally required; however, close observation is crucial, as pulpal necrosis can develop later, requiring endodontic intervention.[62]

When an immature tooth is intruded up to 7 mm, observation for spontaneous re-eruption over three weeks is recommended. If no movement occurs, orthodontic repositioning should be initiated. For intrusions exceeding 7 mm, surgical or orthodontic repositioning should be performed within three weeks. In teeth with closed apices, limited intrusion (<3 mm) in patients under 17 years may still result in spontaneous reeruption. If the tooth fails to re-erupt within two to three weeks, orthodontic extrusion or, in severe cases, extraction followed by reimplantation may be required.[62]

A key risk associated with intrusive luxation is ankylosis, where the tooth becomes fused to the alveolar bone, often resulting in infraposition. Once ankylosis develops, tooth movement becomes difficult or impossible except through surgical intervention. Patients should be informed that the long-term prognosis of intruded teeth is uncertain, as eventual tooth loss due to ankylosis is a common outcome.[62]

Splinting of luxated teeth should only be carried out when the tooth remains mobile after repositioning, using a flexible splint that permits physiological movement of the tooth during healing. In evaluating luxation trauma, the stage of root development must be considered:

In teeth with open apices, pulpal revascularization is often possible, allowing continued root development.

In teeth with closed apices, pulpal necrosis is more likely, necessitating endodontic treatment.[62]

If the apex is closed, endodontic treatment is likely needed. It is advisable to follow the patient closely or refer him or her to an endodontist for further evaluation. Because of the injury to the PDL, rapid inflammatory root resorption can occur (within days or a few weeks) if the necrotic pulpal tissue becomes infected. For mature teeth diagnosed with necrotic pulps, placing calcium hydroxide for two to four weeks prior to obturation is recommended; however, one should allow the PDL to heal for two weeks before placement (see treatment for avulsion below). Apexification or revascularization is recommended for teeth with open apices.[62]

Avulsion

The extra-alveolar time of an avulsed tooth is the most critical determinant of its prognosis. When the tooth is replanted within 30 minutes, the likelihood of periodontal ligament (PDL) survival and successful healing is high. Alternatively, if immediate replantation is not possible, storing the tooth in a physiological medium, such as Hank's Balanced Salt Solution (HBSS) or milk, for a few hours can help preserve PDL cell viability. However, if the tooth remains dry for more than one hour, the PDL cells are irreversibly damaged, and ankylosis is the most likely long-term outcome. Once the tooth has been replanted, physiological splinting for approximately two weeks is recommended to provide stability during the healing period.[66]

In contrast, when a tooth with a closed apex is avulsed, revascularization is not expected. Therefore, root canal treatment should be started approximately two weeks after replantation, ideally before the splint is removed. Beginning treatment earlier than this is not advised, as excessive manipulation during or immediately after replantation may exacerbate PDL injury.[66]

In the case of a closed apex, revascularization is not expected. Therefore, endodontic treatment must be initiated two weeks after the tooth is reimplanted, and prior to removal of the splint. Treatment should not be initiated earlier as any further manipulation of the tooth prior to or immediately after reimplantation can cause further damage to the PDL.[66]

In addition, it has been shown that placing calcium hydroxide as an intracanal medicament immediately after reimplantation will promote inflammation that can lead to PDL damage. If the tooth had been kept dry longer than 60 minutes, performing root canal treatment prior to replantation is indicated.[66]

After managing the emergency phase and stabilizing the tooth, the second stage of treatment involves long-term monitoring of the pulpal status and the potential for root resorption. Regular follow-up examinations over several months are essential to evaluate healing and detect any pathological changes early.[66]

Traumatic dental injuries continue to pose complex clinical challenges for both practitioners and patients. However, advances in evidence-based management have made it possible to achieve highly favorable outcomes in cases that previously resulted in tooth loss or significant esthetic compromise. Through timely diagnosis, appropriate emergency care, and consistent follow-up, clinicians can often convert a seemingly hopeless situation into a successful functional and esthetic result. The endodontic specialist plays a central role within the multidisciplinary team, ensuring that both the pulpal and periradicular tissues are preserved or restored to health following trauma.[66]

IATROGENIC FACTORS CAUSING ENDODONTIC EMERGENCY

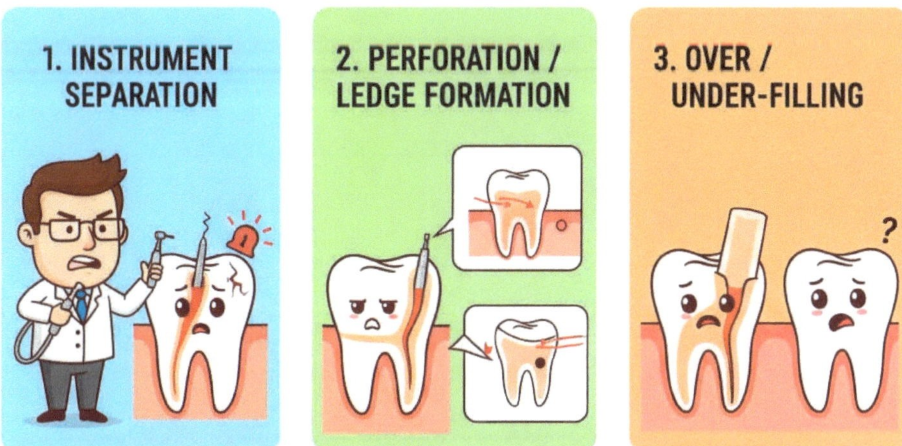

PREVENTABLE ERRORS REQUIRING URGENT CARE!

IATROGENIC FACTORS CAUSING ENDODONTIC EMERGENCY

Deep dental caries often provoke a strong inflammatory response within the dental pulp, which, if left unchecked, may progress to pulpal necrosis. During the excavation of deep carious lesions, the protective dentin barrier covering the pulp can be inadvertently compromised, thereby impairing the pulp's natural healing capacity. To minimize this risk, research has shown that employing a stepwise caries excavation technique, rather than complete removal of caries in a single visit, reduces the likelihood of pulp exposure and promotes favorable pulpal healing. The pulpal response to dental treatment is influenced by multiple factors, including thermal injury, mechanical trauma to odontoblastic processes, desiccation of dentin, vibration, pulp exposure, formation of a smear layer, remaining dentin thickness, the type of restorative material used, and the extent of microleakage following restoration. Thermal injury is a major concern during cavity preparation. The use of rotary cutting instruments, such as burs or stones, generates significant frictional heat, which can adversely affect pulpal health. The degree of intrapulpal temperature rise depends on various factors, including the rotational speed of the bur, the size, type, and shape of the cutting instrument, the duration of contact with the dentin, the pressure applied on the handpiece, the cutting technique employed, and the use or absence of coolant. Adequate water spray and intermittent cutting are therefore essential to prevent excessive heat buildup and safeguard pulpal vitality.[67]

Studies have shown that high-speed cutting with copious water coolant and a reduced force results in minimal histological alteration of the pulp. Magnusson & Sundell found an advantage of stepwise excavation: only 15% of the pulps were exposed compared with 53% after complete excavation.[68] Similar findings were reported by Leksell et al (18% vs. 40%).[69]

Wittrock et al. have demonstrated that cutting technique used during cavity preparation plays a critical role in the amount of heat generated within the tooth. When tooth preparation is carried out in close proximity to the pulp, excessive frictional heat may be produced, leading to a marked rise in intrapulpal temperature that can adversely affect pulp vitality. Such thermal injury has been associated with irreversible pulpal damage if adequate cooling is not maintained. Clinical follow-ups of teeth restored with cast restorations (full crowns and teeth included as abutments in bridgework) have shown that pulpal necrosis may occur with a frequency of 10-15% over a period of 5-10 years.[70]

Another complication to cavity and crown preparation is internal bleeding. In rare cases it may be so extensive that pulpal necrosis occurs almost instantaneously. The tooth structure of such teeth may turn red and later a grey colour.[71]

Injury to odontoblasts: Odontoblasts are continuously exposed to a range of mechanical, thermal, and chemical insults, including frictional heat, amputation of odontoblastic processes, cell body displacement, vibration, and exposure to bacterial toxins or other chemical irritants. These cells are closely packed, interconnected by permanent and transient junctions, which maintain the integrity and spacing of the odontoblastic layer. This structural arrangement regulates the movement of molecules and tissue fluids between the dentin and the pulp, playing a key role in pulpal homeostasis. Routine dental procedures can temporarily disrupt the odontoblastic layer and, in some cases, may cause permanent cellular injury. During cavity preparation, odontoblastic processes may be amputated at various points along their distal segments depending on the depth of the cavity. If the processes are not severed near the cell body, the cell membrane can repair itself and the odontoblast survives. However, if the odontoblasts die, they undergo autolysis and are subsequently replaced by new odontoblast-like cells derived from odontogenic progenitor cells. This regenerative process is successful only if the underlying cell-rich zone of the pulp remains intact and uninjured, preserving the pulp's capacity for repair and continued dentin formation.[71]

Desiccation of dentine: Prolonged use of compressed air to dry a cavity can delay pulpal healing. Rapid evaporation of dentinal fluids generates strong capillary forces, stimulating mechanoreceptors that may cause postoperative pain and displacement of odontoblasts along the tubules. Displaced cells undergo autolysis, but are replaced by cells from the underlying uninjured pulp. Vigorous drying alone does not cause major irreversible pulpal damage. Degradation products are diluted by dentinal fluid, and too few cells are affected to trigger significant inflammation. Over 1–3 months, tertiary (reparative) dentin is deposited to protect the pulp at the site of injury.[71]

Vibration: The impact of vibratory forces from cutting burs on the pulp has not been extensively studied. According to Holden, shock waves generated by the bur propagate beneath the point of contact in the pulp. These effects are amplified when the bur is stalled by digital pressure, which not only reduces cutting efficiency due to clogging but also increases intrapulpal temperature, potentially contributing to pulpal injury.[71]

Pulp exposure: Pulp exposure most commonly occurs during removal of deep carious dentin or placement of pins and retention points. Friction-locked pins may produce microfractures, creating a pathway between dentin and pulp. In such cases, the pulp is primarily affected by bacterial contamination. Studies by Frank demonstrated that pulps exposed in germ-free rats healed completely without any inflammatory response, highlighting the central role of microbial invasion in pulpal injury.[71]

Secondary Factors Result in Pulp Injury

Smear Layer: Rotary instrumentation produces an amorphous layer of microcrystalline debris on enamel and dentin, known as the smear layer. Its management is debated. One view suggests that the smear layer occludes dentinal tubules, reducing permeability and limiting bacterial ingress. However, Pashley argued that bacterial toxins and by-products can still penetrate and cause pulpal inflammation. Brännström noted that most restorative materials do not bond well to dentin, allowing bacteria from the smear layer to infiltrate contraction gaps and compromise the pulp.[71]

Microleakage: Despite advances in restorative materials and placement techniques, polymerization shrinkage of resin composites remains a concern. Shrinkage generates stress within the restoration, potentially creating gaps at the tooth–restoration interface. These gaps allow bacteria and their by-products to penetrate toward the pulp, causing pulpal irritation, a phenomenon referred to as microleakage.[71]

Recent research shows that bacterial leakage at restoration margins poses a significant threat to pulp vitality, especially in deep or extensive dentin exposures. Pulpal inflammation in this context resembles that seen in caries, but the response is often more acute due to the sudden bacterial load. Neutrophils play a key role in the initial defense, accumulating in pulp regions corresponding to affected dentinal tubules and migrating in response to chemotactic signals. Along with the protective effects of dentinal fluid, this response helps limit bacterial penetration into the pulp. These mechanisms likely account for why pulpal repair and healing can occur even when a restoration does not achieve a perfect marginal seal.[71]

Toxic Effects of Restorative Material: Beyond the trauma from tooth preparation and bacterial leakage, constituents of restorative materials can adversely affect the pulp. Historically, material toxicity was considered a major cause of pulpal injury. Contributing factors include chemical cytotoxicity, exothermic reactions during setting, acidity, water absorption during polymerization, and poor marginal adaptation, which can lead to microleakage and secondary pulpal irritation.[71]

Recent research indicates that toxic components of restorative materials pose a lesser threat to the pulp than previously thought. Experimental studies applying materials such as amalgam, zinc phosphate cement, and resin composites directly onto pulpal tissue showed that, when the restoration surface was sealed bacteria-tight, the pulp often returned to a healthy state. In contrast, without a proper seal, severe pulpal inflammation developed. The presence of a dentin barrier further reduces risk, acting as a detoxifying tissue by absorbing harmful substances within dentinal tubules and buffering the effects of acids and bases.[71]

Both in vitro and in vivo studies indicate that the penetration and cytotoxicity of resin monomers—such as triethylene glycol dimethacrylate (TEGDMA) and 2-hydroxyethyl methacrylate (HEMA)—into the pulp are not fully understood. Animal studies suggest that any toxic effects are short-lived. Most leachable substances from resin composites are released within the first few days after placement, with minimal subsequent discharge. Consequently, pulpal risk from restorative procedures arises primarily from an inadequate marginal seal, rather than from the material itself.[71]

In addition, the exothermic reaction of some luting cements on setting has been thought to cause pulpal injury. However, Plant (1976) demonstrated that zinc phosphate, the most exothermic cement, caused an intrapulpal increase in temperature of just 2°C. This is insufficient to cause any injury to the pulp. Changing the amount of powder and liquid ratios when mixing cements however was shown to cause a marked rise in temperature.[71]

Remaining dentine thickness: Over time, the required remaining dentin thickness (RDT) to maintain pulp health has been reconsidered. Stanley suggested that 2 mm of RDT is needed to protect the pulp during most restorative procedures. Pameijer reported that 1 mm or more is sufficient to shield the pulp from the cytotoxic effects of zinc phosphate and resin-modified glass ionomer cements during luting. Murray observed that cavities cut to 0.5 mm depth had only a limited impact on odontoblast survival, indicating that careful preparation can preserve pulpal health even in deeper cavities.[71]

Root Planning: Pulpal response to root planing is generally negligible, provided dentin removal is limited. Exposed dentinal tubules can heal and repair even in the presence of microorganisms, depending on the remaining dentin thickness. However, if periodontal involvement reaches the apical foramen, curettage may sever pulp blood vessels, leading to pulpal damage, and prophylactic root canal treatment is often indicated. In summary, unless the root apex is involved, periodontal therapy has minimal impact on the pulp.[71]

Local Anaesthetics: Although intra-ligamentary injections have been suggested as a cause of pulpal damage, both clinical and animal studies show no adverse effects on the pulp. Physiologic changes, such as a rapid and marked reduction in pulpal blood flow due to adrenaline, do occur, but these vascular alterations do not appear to harm the pulp, even when combined with restorative procedures.[71]

Electrosurgery: Electrosurgery, used to remove gingival tissue for improved access during tooth preparation or impressions, can affect the pulp if the probe contacts a metallic restoration. Adverse pulpal reactions occur with both metallic and non-metallic restorations, and severity increases with longer contact time and reduced remaining dentin thickness (RDT). Contact exceeding 0.4 seconds has been shown to cause irreversible pulpal damage.[71]

Bleaching of Vital Teeth: Vital teeth can be bleached using in-office or at-home techniques. In-office bleaching typically involves applying a high-concentration hydrogen peroxide gel (≈35%) to teeth isolated with a rubber dam. Activation with heat or light may be employed to enhance the oxidizing effect of the peroxide and improve bleaching efficacy. [71]

At-home bleaching typically uses a 10% carbamide peroxide solution applied in a custom-fitted tray worn by the patient, often overnight. Although peroxide can penetrate to the pulp, causing transient sensitivity, studies show that the pulp remains healthy and any sensitivity is fully reversible.[71]

The rate of oxygen release from bleaching agents, and thus the speed of colour change, is temperature-dependent, with a 10 °C increase approximately doubling the reaction rate. However, excessive heat can cause tooth sensitivity or irreversible pulpal inflammation. Bleaching should be performed without anaesthesia to prevent overheating. As many operative procedures are traumatic to the pulp, their effects can be cumulative.[71]

Dental practitioners must be fully aware of procedures and materials that may compromise the pulp. Proper cavity preparation and careful technique can significantly reduce pulpal injury. Materials such as cavity varnishes, liners, and bases are widely used to protect the pulp. Other factors influencing pulpal prognosis include patient-related aspects such as age, previous dental treatment, tooth characteristics, and diet, which can all affect healing and long-term pulp health.[71]

INTER-APPOINTMENT EMERGENCIES

1. ENDONOTIC FLARE-UP

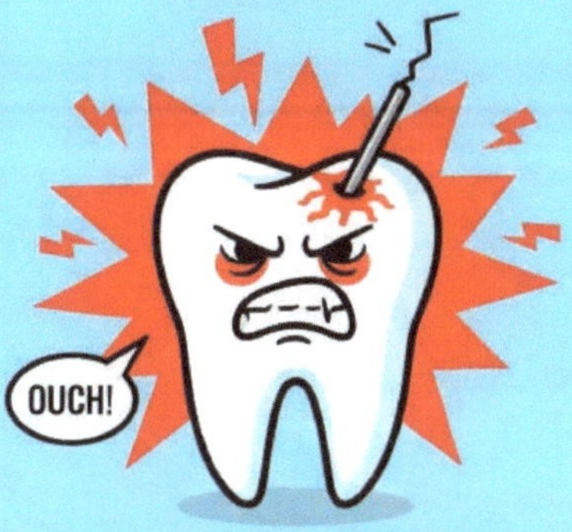

- Pain between appoinments
- Suden, severe onset
- History of root canal treatment

2. RECENT RESTORATIVE TREATMENT

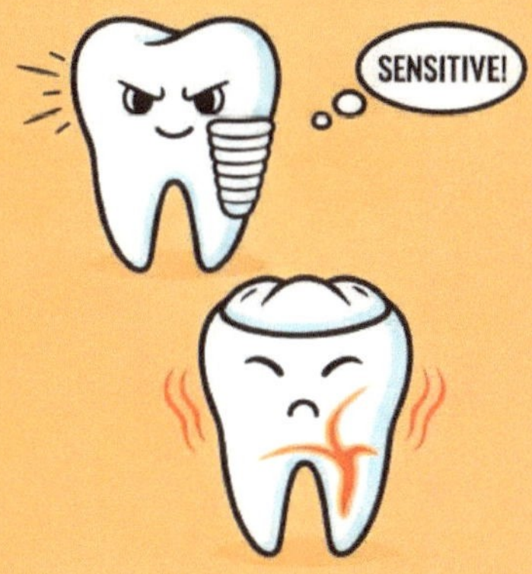

- Pain after new filling/crown
- Sensitivity to hot/cold
- Bite feels 'off

UNXEXPECTED PAIN REQUIRING URGENT DENTAL VISIT!

INTER-APPOINTMENT EMERGENCIES

An interappointment flare-up is a true endodontic emergency requiring unscheduled treatment. Despite careful procedures, patients may experience pain, swelling, or temporary regional paresthesia. Such flare-ups are undesirable and disruptive but must be managed promptly. While sometimes unpredictable, their likelihood can often be anticipated based on specific patient factors.[72]

Understanding the causes and mechanisms of interappointment pain is essential for prevention and management. This pain arises from mechanical, chemical, or microbial injury to the pulp or periradicular tissues during root canal treatment. Microorganisms contribute when there is apical extrusion of debris, incomplete instrumentation altering the microbial environment, or secondary intraradicular infections.[73].

Interappointment pain is almost exclusively due to the development of acute inflammation at the periradicular tissues in response to an increase in the intensity of injury coming from the root canal system. When an interappointment emergency occurs, proper diagnosis and active treatment are required for the clinician to succeed in solving the problem. [73]

Definition: A flare-up may be defined as the occurrence of severe pain and/or swelling following an endodontic treatment appointment, requiring an unscheduled visit and active treatment (Walton & Fouad 1992)[72]data were collected at root canal treatment appointments on demographics, pulp/periapical diagnoses, presenting symptoms, treatment procedures, and number of appointments. Patients that then experienced a flare-up (a severe problem requiring an unscheduled visit and treatment.

Even with careful technique, patients may experience pain after endodontic procedures. It is important to inform patients in advance that some discomfort is normal, arising from an inflammatory response at the tooth apex. For mild pain, over-the-counter analgesics, preferably NSAIDs, are recommended. Persistent pain beyond two to three days may indicate the need for further evaluation and treatment, which could be due to specific underlying causes.[74]

Incidence

Studies report a low overall incidence of interappointment flare-ups, ranging from 1.4% to 3% (Mor et al., 1992). Variations in reported rates may result from differences in study design, patient populations, clinical conditions, and outcome criteria. Many earlier studies were retrospective, uncontrolled, or involved small sample sizes, limiting their reliability. Well-controlled prospective studies confirm that flare-ups are generally uncommon, and most postoperative discomfort is mild, though incidence can vary under certain clinical circumstances.[76]

Mild postoperative pain is relatively common, even when endodontic treatment adheres to accepted standards. Following chemo-mechanical preparation, 10–30% of patients may experience mild discomfort, which is generally tolerable or managed effectively with common analgesics. In contrast, the development of moderate to severe interappointment pain, with or without swelling, is uncommon and represents an unusual clinical scenario.[77]

Several factors can significantly affect the development of interappointment pain, including patient age, gender, tooth type, pulpal status, preoperative pain, allergies, and the presence of a sinus tract. In addition, psychological factors such as dental anxiety, fear, and apprehension may influence pain perception and individual reaction thresholds, highlighting the importance of considering both clinical and patient-related variables in endodontic care.[79]

Studies have shown an association between preoperative apprehension and the development of postoperative pain. Understanding the causes and mechanisms of interappointment pain is essential for the clinician to prevent or manage this complication effectively. When an interappointment emergency occurs, accurate diagnosis and prompt, active treatment are critical for resolving the problem successfully.[80]

- The two conditions that may require emergency treatment during a course of root canal treatment are[80]:
  - **Endodontic flare up**
  - **Recent restorative treatment**

7.1 ENDODONTIC FLARE-UPS

Causes of interappointment pain

Interappointment pain arises from mechanical, chemical, or microbial injury to the pulp or periradicular tissues, often exacerbated during root canal treatment. Regardless of the injury type, the intensity of the inflammatory response is generally proportional to the degree of tissue damage. As vascular events associated with acute inflammation typically produce pain, it follows that more intense inflammatory reactions tend to cause greater pain, although other patient- and procedure-related factors may also influence pain perception.[81,87]

While mechanical and chemical injuries are often linked to iatrogenic factors, microbial injury remains the most common and significant cause of interappointment pain. Studies indicate that the incidence of pain is notably higher in teeth with periradicular lesions compared to teeth with vital pulps and healthy periradicular tissues, highlighting the critical role of infection control in endodontic treatment.[81]

Microbial involvement can play a role in pain causation even when root canal procedures have been performed judiciously and carefully.

Microbial causes

Certain circumstances can predispose teeth to microbial-induced interappointment pain. In most cases, pain arises from an imbalance in the host–bacteria relationship triggered by intracanal procedures. The development of pain due to infectious agents depends on multiple, often interconnected factors, including the extent of microbial contamination, host immune response, and procedural variables, emphasizing the complex interplay between infection and pulpal or periradicular tissue response. [81,87]

- **Presence of pathogenic bacteria**
- **Presence of virulent clonal types**
- **Microbial synergism**
- **Number of microbial cells**
- **Environmental casts**
- **Host resistance**

- **Herpesvirus infection**
    - Apical extrusion of debris
    - Incomplete instrumentation
    - Secondary intraradicular infections
- **Non-microbial causes**

Presence of pathogenic bacteria

The progression of periradicular disease from an asymptomatic to symptomatic state is not well documented. Consequently, there is limited evidence regarding qualitative or quantitative shifts in the endodontic microbiota that may accompany or trigger exacerbations, making it challenging to identify the bacterial species responsible for symptomatic infections. Evidence suggests that certain bacteria are frequently associated with symptomatic periradicular lesions, including Porphyromonas endodontalis, Porphyromonas gingivalis, Prevotella species, Treponema denticola, Tannerella forsythia, Filifactor alocis, Dialister pneumosintes, Peptostreptococcus micros, and Finegoldia magna. Recent studies indicate that Fusobacterium nucleatum, Prevotella, and Porphyromonas species are often isolated in flare-up cases, suggesting that the bacteria involved in flare-ups may be similar to those in primarily infected root canals with symptomatic periradicular lesions. Interestingly, several studies have found that bacteria present in asymptomatic cases can also predispose teeth to flare-ups, highlighting the complex and sometimes unpredictable nature of endodontic infections. [81,85,86]

Presence of virulent clonal types

Different clonal types of the same pathogenic bacterial species can vary significantly in their virulence. Consequently, disease attributed to a particular species is often caused by specific virulent clones. The presence of these virulent clones in the root canal may therefore serve as a predisposing factor for interappointment pain, highlighting the importance of microbial composition and pathogenicity in endodontic outcomes.[81]

Microbial Synergism

Many endodontic pathogens exhibit virulence primarily when associated with other microbial species. These synergistic or additive interactions can enhance pathogenicity, influencing the severity of infection and contributing to the development of symptoms, including interappointment pain.[81]

Number of Microbial Cells

The microbial load is a key factor in the pathogenicity of endodontic infections. When the host encounters a higher than usual number of microbial cells, an acute exacerbation of a periradicular lesion may occur. Such increases in microbial load can be accidentally precipitated by endodontic procedures, highlighting the importance of careful canal instrumentation and disinfection.[81]

Environmental Cues

A virulent clone of a pathogenic species does not always express its virulence factors continuously. Evidence indicates that the environment plays a crucial role in switching microbial virulence genes on or off. Studies have shown that environmental changes can influence the behavior of several putative oral and endodontic pathogens, including Porphyromonas gingivalis, Fusobacterium nucleatum, Prevotella intermedia, and oral treponemes. If intracanal procedures alter the root canal environment in a way that favors virulence gene expression, microbial pathogenicity can increase, potentially leading to interappointment pain.[81]

Host Resistance

Host resistance is a critical factor in determining whether an infection will progress to disease. Individuals vary in their ability to resist infections, and these differences can become evident over a lifetime. Hypothetically, patients with reduced immune competence may be more likely to develop clinical symptoms, including interappointment pain, following endodontic procedures in infected root canals.[81]

Herpes Virus Infection

Viral infections can further compromise host resistance, potentially exacerbating interappointment pain. Herpes viruses, for example, can interfere with the host immune response, promoting the overgrowth of pathogenic bacteria and reducing the host's ability to control infection. Additionally, these viruses may stimulate the release of proinflammatory cytokines from host defense cells. Recent studies have shown that active infections of periradicular lesions by human cytomegalovirus or Epstein–Barr virus are significantly associated with symptomatic manifestations.[82]

The possibility exists that active herpes virus infections in periradicular lesions may initiate or contribute to flare-ups. The mechanisms behind herpes viruses' involvement with symptomatic periradicular lesions remain elusive.[82]

There are some situations during the endodontic treatment that can facilitate microorganisms to cause inter-appointment pain. These include: [81]

A. **Apical extrusion of debris.**

B. **Incomplete instrumentation leading to changes in the endodontic microbiota or in environmental conditions.**

C. **Secondary intraradicular infections.**

A. **Apical extrusion of debris:** Extrusion of infected debris into the periradicular tissues during chemo-mechanical preparation is considered a major cause of postoperative pain. In asymptomatic teeth with periradicular lesions, a balance exists between the microbial challenge from the endodontic microbiota and the host defenses in the periradicular tissues. When microorganisms are inadvertently extruded beyond the apex, the host is confronted with an increased microbial load, disrupting this balance. This triggers a transient acute inflammatory response as the host attempts to restore equilibrium, often resulting in postoperative discomfort.[81]

The risks of interappointment pain during the treatment of infected cases can be even higher in the event of over instrumentation. In those cases, exacerbations caused by iatrogenic over instrumentation are likely to develop as a result of mechanical injury to the periradicular tissues, which is usually coupled with apical extrusion of a significant number of debris containing microorganisms.[81]

Forcing microorganisms and their products into the periradicular tissues can generate an acute inflammatory response, whose intensity will depend on the number and/or virulence of the extruded microorganisms.[81]

The development of postoperative pain is influenced by both quantitative and qualitative factors. The quantitative factor refers to the number of microbial cells extruded into the periradicular tissues, while the qualitative factor relates to the virulence of the extruded microorganisms. All root canal instrumentation techniques result in some apical extrusion of debris, but the amount varies significantly among techniques. Greater debris extrusion is associated with a higher risk of postoperative pain. Crown-down techniques, whether performed with hand or engine-driven instruments, generally extrude less debris and are therefore preferred for the instrumentation of infected root canals.[81]

The quantitative factor the number of extruded microbial cells is largely under the clinician's control through careful instrumentation. In contrast, the qualitative factor, which relates to the virulence of the bacteria, is more difficult to manage. When virulent clonal types of pathogenic bacteria are present in the root canal and are pushed into the periradicular tissues during instrumentation, even a small volume of infected debris can trigger or exacerbate periradicular inflammation, potentially leading to postoperative or interappointment pain.[81]

B. **Incomplete instrumentation:** The microbiota of primary endodontic infections usually exists as a mixed microbial consortium, where alterations in one portion of the community can affect both the environment and the remaining species. Potent exogenous forces, such as chemomechanical preparation with antimicrobial irrigants and intracanal medications, are required to effectively eradicate these microbial communities. However, incomplete chemomechanical preparation can disrupt the microbial balance by eliminating some inhibitory species while leaving others unchecked, allowing them to overgrow. If the overgrown strains are virulent and/or numerically dominant, they can intensify periradicular tissue damage and precipitate lesion exacerbation.

Environmental changes induced by incomplete instrumentation can also activate microbial virulence genes, potentially converting a previously asymptomatic case into a symptomatic one. Another proposed environmental factor is the entrance of oxygen into the root canal, which may alter the oxidation–reduction potential (Eh), theoretically promoting a shift from anaerobic to facultative bacterial growth and acute periradicular inflammation. However, this Oxygen–Eh theory remains speculative, as scientific evidence supporting it is lacking.[81]

C. **Secondary intraradicular infections:** Secondary intraradicular infections arise from microorganisms that were absent in the primary infection and gain access to the root canal during treatment, between appointments, or even after completion of endodontic therapy. The most common route of entry is a breach of the aseptic chain during treatment. If these microorganisms survive and colonize the root canal, a secondary infection may develop. When the newly established microbial species are virulent and reach sufficient numbers, they can trigger acute periradicular inflammation, potentially causing postoperative or interappointment pain.[81]

Non-Microbial Causes

Microorganisms are essential for the induction and perpetuation of periradicular diseases, as they provide a persistent source of irritation. However, non-microbial factors can also provoke periradicular inflammation, although such inflammation is usually transient unless it coincides with microbial aggression. Despite being temporary, inflammation caused by chemical or physical insults can still result in pain. The intensity of this pain depends on several factors, including the nature and extent of the tissue insult, proximity to the apex, and the host's inflammatory response.[81]

- **Intensity of the injury.**
- **Intensity of tissue damage.**
- **Intensity of the inflammatory response.**

When instruments, irrigants, medications, and filling materials are confined to the interior of the root canal, the risk of pain from physical or chemical injury is generally low. Non-microbial causes of periradicular inflammation are often iatrogenic. Mechanical irritation may occur from over-instrumentation or overextended filling materials. In over-instrumentation, larger instruments inflict more damage to periradicular tissues, triggering a more intense inflammatory response and increasing the likelihood of postoperative pain. Over-instrumentation is often accompanied by extrusion of infected debris. Overextended filling materials can mechanically compress periradicular tissues, inducing pain.

Chemical irritation can result from the apical extrusion of irrigants or intracanal medications, which are cytotoxic to host tissues. Despite this, clinical trials indicate that proper use of these substances rarely affects postoperative symptoms. Endodontic sealers are also cytotoxic prior to setting, and overextension of these materials increases tissue injury. Larger amounts of overfilled sealer correlate with higher intensity of periradicular damage, and thus significantly increase the risk of postoperative pain.[81]

Inflammatory Events Leading to Interappointment Pain

Interappointment pain is almost exclusively due to the development of acute inflammation at the periradicular tissues in response to an increase in the intensity of injury coming from the root canal system. The inflammatory response to tissue injury can be regarded as a double-edged sword.[81]

On the one hand, it provides protection against infection and/or prepares the injured area for repair of the tissue architecture. On the other hand, inflammatory reaction can result in undesirable effects such as pain and intensified tissue damage.[81]

As previously mentioned, microorganisms are the major causative agents of periradicular inflammation. Whatever the mechanisms by which microorganisms are involved, interappointment pain is a result of acute periradicular inflammation in response to a sudden increase in the amount of microbial irritants. The host is challenged by a higher number of microbial cells and/or products than it was used to coping with the balance between aggression and defense. The host mounts an acute inflammatory reaction at the periradicular tissues in an attempt to re-establish the equilibrium. Chemical mediators released after tissue injury can directly lower the excitability threshold of the sensory nerve fibers, can induce pain due to direct effect on the nerve fibers, or can cause pain indirectly by inducing increase of the vascular permeability, which produces edema and swelling.[81]

In the majority of circumstances in which interappointment pain is caused by microorganisms, an infection is established in the root canal system and the periradicular tissues are usually chronically inflamed.[81]

Bacteria that suddenly gain access to the periradicular tissues are faced with two immediate lines of defense, represented by the complement system and by phagocytes (neutrophils and macrophages) present in the chronically inflamed tissue. Bacteria may be recognized directly and engulfed by neutrophils and macrophages with receptors for common bacterial components. [81]

The activation of complement by the classic, alternative or lectin pathways and the engulfment of bacteria by phagocytes can occur in the early hours of host-pathogen interaction in an already inflamed tissue. The encounter of the bacteria with these host defense mechanisms triggers the production and release of chemical mediators of inflammation, which will induce vascular changes in the microcirculation and recruit new phagocytic cells to the site.[83,92]

When bacterial mass comes into contact with the periradicular tissues, it may carry a high load of virulence factors that diffuse through tissues and stimulate host defenses. These factors include cellular components such as lipopolysaccharide, peptidoglycan, lipoteichoic acid, and fimbriae, metabolic byproducts like butyrate, propionate, and sulfur compounds, and peptides containing

N-formyl-methionine-leucyl-phenylalanine. Such bacterial constituents can activate macrophages and also trigger the complement system via the alternative pathway, amplifying the local inflammatory response.[83,92]

Bacterial metabolic end products are toxic to host tissues and can stimulate the release of pro-inflammatory cytokines, contributing to periradicular inflammation. N-formylmethionine-leucyl-phenylalanine (N-fMLP) peptides act as chemoattractants for neutrophils, allowing these immune cells to detect bacterial proteins. Only bacterial proteins and a few mitochondrially synthesized mammalian proteins are initiated by fMLP. Phagocytic cells, including neutrophils, are strategically located at sites of potential microbial entry. In infected root canals, phagocytes accumulate near the apical foramen, forming a defense to prevent bacterial invasion into the periradicular tissues.[83]

In response to bacterial challenge, phagocytes can release a variety of mediators, such as cytokines (IL-1, IL-6, IL-8, IL-12, TNF-a), prostaglandins, oxygenderived radicals, leukotrienes (particularly LTB4), and platelet-activating factor (PAF).[84]

These products of phagocytes, the activation of the complement system by any of the three pathways generates mediators such as:[84]

- **C5a and C3a: C5a is a powerful chemotactic agent for neutrophils and monocytes.**
- **Activation of mast cells followed by release of histamine: Histamine causes dilation of arterioles and increases permeability of venules.**

The combined local effects of these mediators result in exacerbation of the inflammatory response, which usually starts immediately after increase in bacterial aggression and may take some hours before signs and symptoms become evident.[84]

The inflammatory exudate leaving the vessels and accumulating in tissues will elevate the tissue hydrostatic pressure, which results in swelling and pain. Endothelium usually becomes leaky in inflammation due to:85

- Formation of gaps between endothelial cells in venules, which is elicited by mediators such as histamine, bradykinin, leukotrienes, PAF, and substance P.
- Direct endothelial cell injury induced by direct damage to the endothelium by the injurious agent.
- Endothelium injury mediated by leukocytes which adhere to endothelium early in inflammation and, if activated in the process, they can release oxygen radicals and lysosomal enzymes, causing endothelial injury

Certain inflammatory mediators can induce pain by directly stimulating sensory nerve fibers. Additionally, the exudation of fluid into tissues increases hydrostatic pressure, compressing nerve endings and is considered a major factor in pain associated with acute inflammation. Elevated tissue pressure can also distend soft tissues, resulting in swelling. The increased hydrostatic pressure is therefore central to pain of endodontic origin. The guiding principle in emergency management of such cases is the drainage of exudate to relieve tissue pressure and rapidly alleviate pain.[85]

Macrophages, in response to bacterial stimuli, secrete IL-1 and TNF, which stimulate endothelial cells to express molecules that facilitate the selective attachment and migration of leukocytes. Bacterial products, such as lipopolysaccharide (LPS), can similarly activate endothelial cells, producing changes akin to those induced by TNF. Polymorphonuclear neutrophils are the first leukocytes to arrive at the site of injury. When exposed to IL-8 and TNF-α, neutrophils become activated, generating a respiratory burst that produces oxygen radicals and releasing granule contents, aiding in bacterial elimination.

However, when neutrophils and macrophages are strongly activated, tissue damage may occur, as oxygen radicals and lysosomal enzymes cannot distinguish between host tissues and bacteria. This extreme tissue injury can result in abscess formation. Among the proteolytic enzymes in neutrophil granules, elastase, collagenase, and gelatinase are particularly potent in degrading components of the extracellular matrix, contributing to connective tissue destruction.[83]

Further metabolic and membrane perturbations that occur in neutrophils during chemotaxis, activation, and phagocytosis result in the release of products not only within the phagolysosome, but also potentially in the extracellular environment.[85]

- **The ways by which lysosomal enzymes can be released from neutrophils are the following:**

1. **Death of the cell, resulting in leakage of enzymes into the surrounding tissues.**
2. **Lysis of the cell induced by bacterial products.**
    a. **Fusion of the lysosome with phagocytic vacuoles before the vacuoles have been completely formed resulting in leakage of the enzymes.**
3. **Discharge of lysosomal enzymes into the medium when the cell is brought into contact with targets difficult to be ingested (large colonies, bacteria adhered to flat surfaces, etc.)**

Periradicular inflammation is not solely caused by microorganisms; physical and chemical insults during chemomechanical preparation can also damage periradicular connective tissues. Such insults may trigger mast cell degranulation, leading to the release of histamine into the periradicular tissues. Additionally, vascular injury in the periradicular region can activate cascades mediated by the Hageman factor. When blood vessel damage exposes this factor to negatively charged surfaces, such as collagen and basement membranes, it becomes activated, further contributing to inflammatory responses.[83]

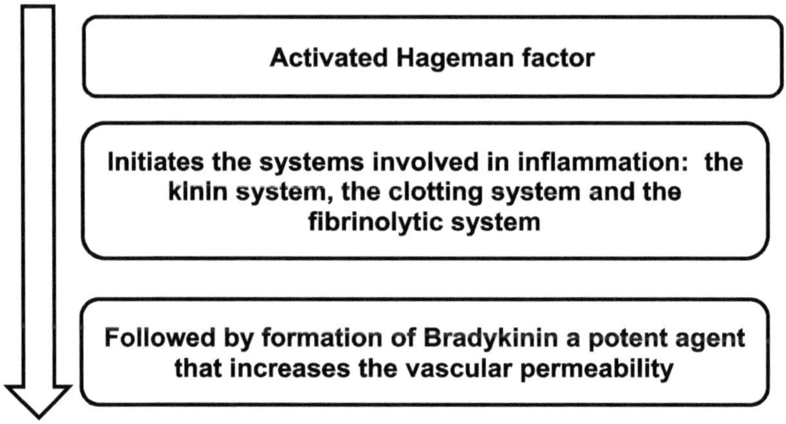

Activation of the clotting system leads to thrombin formation, which cleaves circulating fibrinogen to generate a fibrin clot. During this process, fibrinopeptides are released, increasing vascular permeability and acting as chemoattractants for leukocytes. Activation of the fibrinolytic system produces plasmin, which degrades fibrin into fibrin degradation products that further enhance vascular permeability. Collectively, the activation of these systems contributes to acute inflammation, manifesting as swelling and pain.

In addition, cellular injury caused by chemical or physical factors can release arachidonic acid metabolites, including prostaglandins and leukotrienes, which increase vascular permeability and promote leukocyte chemotaxis. Stimulation of sensory nerve fibers can also trigger the release of neuropeptides, such as substance P and calcitonin gene-related peptide, leading to vasodilation and further enhancement of vascular permeability.[85]

A study found a highly significant association between the presence of allergies to various substances (sulfa medication, pollen, dust, and food stuffs) and the frequency of interappointment pain. It was suggested that this association could have been due to immediate hypersensitivity reaction occurring in the periradicular tissues in response to the egress of antigens from the root canal.[85]

In individuals who are prone to allergies, encounter with some protein antigens or chemicals that bind to proteins elicits activation of TH2 cells and IgE production. IgE antibody produced in response to an antigen binds to high-affinity.[85]

Fc receptors expressed on mast cells.

Mast cell activation occurs after binding of the antigen to two or more IgE molecules on the cell surface. The most important mediators released from mast cells are histamine, prostaglandins, leukotrienes, cytokines, and proteases. Histamine and leukotrienes cause increase in vascular permeability while prostaglandins cause vasodilation. Proteases may also cause damage to the local tissues. Cytokines induce local inflammation.[85]

Hypersensitivity reaction develops within minutes to an hour after exposure to antigens to which the host is sensitized, and interappointment pain takes some hours after intervention to occur. Also, the evidence is lacking as to whether this reaction actually occurs in the periradicular tissues and are responsible for interappointment pain.[85]

Treatment of Interappointment Pain

In a prospective clinical study on post-treatment pain, it was found that 21% of the patients reported slight pain, 15% had moderate pain and 7% experienced severe pain. Although some patients may experience some level of pain after root canal treatment, very few experience the 'true' flare-up, which requires an unscheduled office visit and/or the prescribing of analgesics, systemic steroids and antibiotics. Hargreaves and Seltzer 2002 described an integrated approach for the management and control of odontogenic pain. Termed as the '3D' approach for pain control:[85]

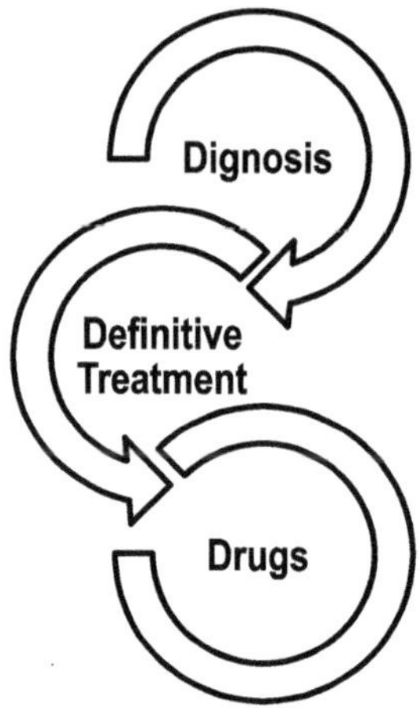

Diagnosis: The first step in managing a patient with post-endodontic pain is an accurate diagnosis. In cases following recent endodontic procedures, diagnosis is often straightforward. However, several conditions can mimic endodontic or odontogenic pain, including issues arising from adjacent teeth, sinus pathology, temporomandibular joint disorders, or post-injection sequelae.

A thorough understanding of the patient's chief complaint is essential. Gathering detailed information—such as onset of symptoms, duration, frequency, intensity, presence of swelling, and factors that exacerbate or relieve the pain—guides the clinician in accurately assessing and managing the situation.[85]

Clinical examination should include percussion (both in axial and right-angle direction), apical palpation, bite-stick challenge, thermal stimulation (cold and hot if indicated) and periodontal probing.[85]

The clinician must decide if taking additional radiographs are indicated. Often times, taking additional, properly angulated radiographs may further elucidate the etiology of the current condition.[85]

Combined clinical and radiographic A thorough clinical examination should then be performed. The following conditions should be properly noted: areas of swelling, discoloration, ulcerations, exudation, defective and/or lost restorations, cracked or fractured tests may reveal that the symptoms are non-odontogenic, are related to another tooth, or related to the recently treated tooth.[85]

Definitive treatment

When a patient presents with endodontic pain, it is important to recognize that they may be experiencing acute physical and emotional distress. Once it is confirmed that the recently treated tooth is the source of the symptoms, prompt and definitive treatment should be provided to alleviate discomfort and address the underlying cause.[85]

A. Re-Instrumentation

Definitive management of a symptomatic tooth may require re-entering the root canal system. Proper anesthesia is essential before any intervention. The access cavity should be reopened, and the tooth anatomy reevaluated, as areas missed during the initial treatment may harbor residual tissue or microorganisms. Use of magnification and illumination enhances visualization and precision during this procedure.

Critical steps include reconfirming working lengths, ensuring apical patency, and thorough debridement with copious irrigation. The primary causes of post-treatment emergencies are residual tissue, microbial contamination, and toxic by-products, sometimes extruded beyond the apex.

In cases of suppurative exudation, allowing drainage through the root canal can relieve localized tissue pressure. There remains some debate on whether teeth should be left open to drain or temporarily sealed to prevent recontamination. Leaving a tooth open may permit reinfection from oral microorganisms, while controlled drainage through enlargement of the apical constriction (to at least a #25 file) has been suggested as a method to relieve exudation. However, studies indicate that trephination through the apex does not always guarantee drainage of periradicular exudate.[85]

B. Cortical Trephination

Cortical trephination involves the surgical perforation of alveolar bone to allow release of accumulated periradicular tissue exudate. Several studies have investigated its effectiveness in preventing or relieving post-treatment pain. Chestner et al. (1968) reported significant pain relief in patients with severe, persistent periradicular pain following cortical trephination. Furthermore, when performed prophylactically in asymptomatic patients, cortical trephination has been shown to reduce the incidence of postoperative pain by 16–25%. Moos et al. (1996) compared postoperative pain outcomes in patients with acute periradicular pain of pulpal origin and found differences between those treated with pulpectomy alone versus pulpectomy combined with cortical trephination.[85]

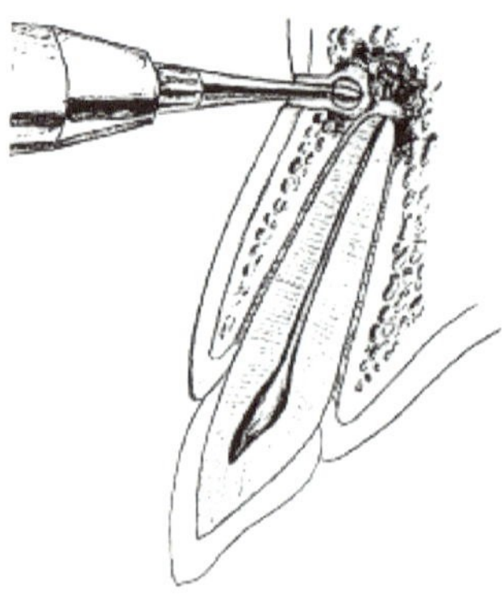

Figure 7: Cortical trephination

Nist et al. 2001 performed a randomized blinded study to evaluate post-operative pain and swelling after performing trephination in symptomatic teeth with periradicular radiolucent lesions. They also found no significant reduction in pain or swelling following the trephination procedure.[85]

C. Incision and Drainage (I&D)

In cases of acute exacerbation of a chronic periradicular lesion or a de novo post-treatment endodontic abscess, establishing drainage through the oral mucosa provides for effective emergency management.[85]

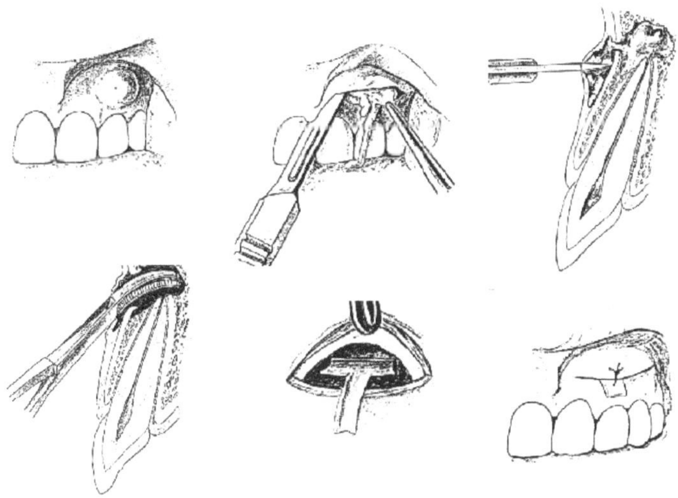

Figure 8: Incision and drainage (I&D)

The primary rationale for an incision and drainage (I&D) procedure is to evacuate pus, microorganisms, and toxic products from the periradicular tissues. This procedure helps to decompress the increased periradicular tissue pressure and provides significant pain relief. In cases where endodontic treatment has not been completed, it may be prudent to re-enter the root canal system to further eliminate the causative factors through debridement, irrigation, and placement of an antimicrobial dressing. Conversely, if the abscess develops after obturation of the root canal system, incision of the fluctuant tissue may be the only feasible emergency intervention.[85]

In cases where root canals are inadequately obturated, it is recommended that the filling material be removed to facilitate additional drainage through the root canal system. Antibiotics may be used to support clinical management in situations of poor drainage, or when the patient presents with concomitant trismus, cellulitis, fever, or lymphadenopathy. Furthermore, aggressive incision and drainage has been advocated for infections associated with cellulitis, regardless of whether the tissue is fluctuant or indurated. Clinical experience indicates that thorough debridement and disinfection of the root canal system, combined with systemic antibiotic therapy, can lead to significant resolution of facial cellulitis associated with endodontic infections.[86]

D. Intracanal Medicaments

Clinical studies have demonstrated that post-treatment pain is neither prevented nor relieved by medicaments such as formocresol, camphorated paramonochlorophenol, eugenol, iodine potassium iodide, Ledermix, or calcium hydroxide.[87]

Studies have shown that use of intracanal steroids, non-steroidal anti-inflammatory drugs (NSAIDs) or a corticosteroid– antibiotic compound has been shown to reduce post-treatment pain[88]. Rogers et al. 1999, demonstrated that both dexamethasone and ketorolac when placed in the root canals of vital teeth after pulpectomy procedures showed statistically significant pain relief at the 12-h time period as compared to the placebo group.[89]

Negm 2001 placed a corticosteroid–antibiotic compound (containing nystatin, neomycin, gramicidin and triamcinolone acetonide in an aqueous cream base), or a placebo (aqueous cream), in the root canals of patients who had returned with post-operative pain following endodontic treatment. It was found that the corticosteroid antibiotic compound was significantly more effective than the placebo in providing pain relief at all time periods up to 24 h.[90] Studies have shown that only steroids and NSAIDs when placed within the root canals system after debridement procedures can reduce or prevent post-treatment pain.[90,90]

F. Occlusal Reduction

The dental literature shows minimal consensus regarding the benefit of occlusal reduction to prevent post-endodontic pain. Studies by Creech et al. and Jostes et al. (1984) indicated that routine occlusal reduction was largely ineffective in preventing postoperative discomfort. In contrast, Rosenberg et al. (1998) demonstrated that in teeth exhibiting pain upon biting, occlusal reduction effectively decreased postoperative pain. Sensitivity to biting and chewing is thought to result from elevated levels of inflammatory mediators stimulating periradicular nociceptors. By reducing occlusal load, the mechanical stimulation of sensitized nociceptors is alleviated, potentially improving patient comfort.[85]

E. Drugs

Antibiotics: In a review on the use of systemic antibiotics for the control of post-treatment endodontic pain, Fouad 2002 concluded that their use is without justification. it appears that antibiotics are frequently prescribed to the patient with endodontic pain. Current advances in our understanding of the biology of the infectious and inflammatory process, along with the known risks associated with antibiotics, such as the emergence of multiresistant bacterial strains, strongly indicate that the clinician should seriously re-evaluate their prescribing habits.[85]

Non-Narcotic Analgesics: Non-narcotic analgesics, NSAIDs and acetaminophen have effectively been used to treat the endodontic pain patient . These drugs produce analgesia by actions in both the peripherally inflamed tissues as well as in certain regions of the brain and spinal cord. The NSAIDs have been shown to be very effective for managing pulpal and periradicular pain. But In patients with known sensitivity to NSAIDs or aspirin, and those who have history of gastrointestinal ulcerations or hypertension due to renal effects of NSAID's, acetominophen should be contraindicated.[91]

The results of several double-blind placebo-controlled trials in endodontic pain patients indicated that 400 mg ibuprofen, 50mg ketoprofen, 100mg flurbiprofen and 30 60mg ketorolac, produce significant analgesia as compared to placebo. Ibuprofen is generally considered the prototype of NSAIDs and has a well-documented efficacy and safety profile. Few endodontic studies showed that comparison of one NSAID with another i.e. 400mg ibuprofen was shown to be similar to 50mg of ketoprofen. Pretreatment with NSAIDs for irreversible pulpitis should have the effect of reducing pulpal and peri radicular levels of the inflammatory mediator PGE2.[92]

The parenteral NSAID ketorolac tromethamine, when injected intraorally or intramuscularly, produced significant analgesia in patients with severe odontogenic pain prior to treatment.[93] Administration of NSAIDs alone is usually sufficient for most endodontic pain patients who can tolerate this drug class. Ibuprofen 600mg taken every 6 h is optimal for managing pulpal and periradicular pain of inflammatory origin. The combination of a NSAID and acetaminophen taken together show additive analgesia for treating dental pain.[91]

7.2 ASPIRATION/SWALLOWING OF DENTAL INSTRUMENTS

Iatrogenic accidents during routine clinical procedures are unpredictable and can occur sometimes regardless of all the possible precautions taken. The golden line "prevention is better than cure" seems to be more of saying and less of a belief when we see cases such as accidental aspiration/swallowing of foreign objects. These foreign objects can be of various sizes and shapes, ranging from small, large, elongated, round, sharp and blunt and can get wedged anywhere either in the gastrointestinal (GI) or the respiratory tract.[94] Webb et al. reported that 92.5% of the swallowed foreign bodies enter the GI tract and 7.5% of these instances in the tracheobronchial tree. Various studies have stated that in all cases reported, only 10–20% cases necessitate nonsurgical intervention, and 1% or less requires surgical retrieval.[95]

Given the high risk of morbidity, costs of specialized care, and potential liability for negligence or malpractice, early recognition and prompt diagnosis of accidental aspiration or ingestion are essential to prevent serious consequences. Delays in proper management and timely intervention can lead to severe complications and, in rare cases, may be fatal. Additionally, such incidents can cause significant emotional distress for patients and their families and may negatively affect a dentist's professional reputation and morale. Therefore, the aim of this review article is to present a case of aspiration of an endodontic broach and to discuss the relevant literature, including risk factors, clinical symptoms, and appropriate management of such iatrogenic incidents. This article also seeks to raise awareness among dental practitioners about the importance of preventive measures and their role in avoiding legal and ethical repercussions.[94]

Incidence

In modern dentistry, patients are generally treated in a supine position to improve visibility, access to the oral cavity, and ergonomic comfort for the operator. While the supine position may increase the risk of accidental aspiration or ingestion of foreign objects, such incidents can occur in any patient position and at any time—not only during treatment but also afterward, as patients handle appliances or prostheses. The incidence of iatrogenic accidents varies widely. Tamura et al., in a review from Japan, reported an incidence ranging from 3.6% to 27.7% of all foreign body cases, with adults showing a higher occurrence than children. Ingestion generally occurs more frequently than aspiration, particularly in children, while children under three years of age are at the highest risk of accidental aspiration, accounting for approximately 80% of cases.[96]

Although any object introduced into the oral cavity can potentially be involved in an accident, some foreign bodies are more frequently ingested or aspirated than others. Dental items are reported as the second most commonly ingested or aspirated objects in adults. Single-tooth cast or prefabricated restorations are particularly prone to aspiration during try-in or cementation. Susini et al. reported that 2.2% of endodontic instruments were aspirated and 18% ingested. Grossman (1991) noted that 87% of ingested endodontic K-files enter the alimentary tract, while 13% reach the respiratory tract. Tiwana et al., in a 10-year institutional review, found that among all dental specialties, fixed prosthodontic treatments had the highest incidence of such accidents, followed by orthodontic procedures.[98]

Etiology / Risk factors

In a healthy state, the larynx acts as a protective sphincter at three different levels at the inlet of the air passage: For aspiration to happen, a foreign object must have to pass these three lines of defense.[94]

- Patients with reduced laryngeal closure are more prone to aspirate saliva, minor dental appliances, instruments or their parts.
- Several patients are at higher risk for aspiration or ingestion. Children aged 1–3 years are at greater risk of swallowing because they chew incompletely with incisors due to the lack of molar eruption and objects or fragments may be propelled posteriorly, triggering a reflex swallow.
- Elderly, IV sedated, inebriated, mentally handicapped, or traumatized patients with altered states of consciousness are usually more susceptible to swallow because of the decreased gag reflex, swallowing incoordination, or other impaired protective airway mechanisms. Sedation decreases both the protective swallowing and cough reflexes. All patients subsequent to cerebrovascular accidents, head trauma, or surgical procedures affecting tongue should be evaluated carefully for aspiration or ingestion due to delayed triggering of swallowing reflex.
- Patients with psychiatric illness, head and neck cancer, and neurologic conditions, such as stroke, dementia, cerebral palsy, brain tumors/injuries, Parkinson's disease, amylotropic lateral sclerosis usually have higher risk due to functional impairment of swallowing mechanism.
- Difficult handling of small slippery (saliva contact) instruments in a limited working region poses an increased risk of aspiration or ingestion and requires special care because of the usual supine or semi-recumbent position of patients. The numbing effect of anesthetic agents and loss of gag reflex mechanism, excessive or unexpected patient

movements during treatment, inadequate lightening, ineffective assistance, limited mouth opening, and unexpected breakage or detachment of poor-quality instruments or its components is also significant contributing factors to aspiration/ingestion of foreign items in dentistry.

- Patients with pregnancy, obesity, and sliding hiatal hernia are also at greater risk of aspiration or ingestion of foreign objects due to increased intra-abdominal pressure, which affects the deglutition reflex resulting in dysphagia, especially in a reclined position.
- Edentulous patients are more susceptible to ingestion of minor items entombed in food bolus due to reduced tactile sensitivity of palate owing to the denture.

Therefore, it is always important to carefully review the patient's medical history during the initial appointment and perform a comprehensive physical examination.

Symptoms Related to Aspiration

Signs and symptoms of aspiration or ingestion differ in conformity with the size and shape of the foreign body and whether it is free, fixed, or perforating.[94]

Aspiration can occur anywhere along the tracheobronchial tree. The right bronchus is usually the most common site in adults because of the anatomic configuration. However, it has been reported in all pulmonary lobes.[94]

- The most common symptoms of laryngotracheal obstruction are dyspnea, cough, and stridor. A laryngeal chocking of the airway by foreign objects results in respiratory difficulty with or without cyanosis and signs of hands clutched to the throat, depending on whether the chocking is partial or complete.

- However, bronchial foreign bodies are associated with cough, decreased air entry, dyspnea, and wheezing. Moreover, some inadvertently aspirated small foreign objects can pass through the vocal cords without obstructing the upper airway and remain asymptomatic for several months
- Their long-term retention can result in late complications such as vocal cord paralysis, postobstructive pneumonia, atelectasis, bronchiectasis, pneumothorax, hemorrhage or lung abscess and death.

Symptoms Related to Ingestion

- In majority of the cases, ingested foreign bodies usually pass through the GI tract uneventfully.
- In case of any obstruction, dysphagia and odynophagia are the most frequently noticed symptoms. However, symptoms such as coughing, gagging, drooling of saliva, chest pain, muscle incoordination, incessant twitching, nausea, hematemesis, and regurgitation may be perceived during esophageal obstruction.
- At potential sites of impaction along the GI tract, the symptoms vary between abdominal pain, fever, nausea, vomiting, and abdominal distension that may complicate diagnosis. Sharp, pointed, and elongated objects such as endodontic reamers and files may fail to pass the fixed curvatures of the duodenum, thereby resulting in impaction or perforation.
- Such perforations can be fatal. Cockerill et al. has reported a case of toothpick ingestion that resulted in death due to a perforation in the third portion of the duodenum and advanced through the inferior vena cava.[94]

Clinical Management of Aspiration/Ingestion Emergencies

Aspiration cases are generally more serious than ingestion and must be treated as emergencies to prevent severe consequences. During an iatrogenic accident, it is crucial for the practitioner to remain calm and composed. The clinician must be able to recognize signs and symptoms of airway or gastric obstruction if a dental item is lost into the oropharynx. The patient should be positioned in a reclined posture and encouraged to cough forcibly to clear the airway. If coughing fails and airway compromise develops, with symptoms such as inspiratory stridor, choking, or labored breathing, the Heimlich maneuver should be performed. If retrieval of the foreign body is not feasible, basic emergency life support should be initiated until definitive intervention can be carried out.[94]

If the airway is not compromised, a prompt assessment for any lost or missing instrument or component should be undertaken, maintaining a high index of suspicion for a mishap. It is therefore essential to carefully examine, explain, and review all equipment used during dental procedures. If the object is located in the oral cavity, it should be immediately retrieved, identified, and checked to ensure it is intact, followed by reassuring the patient. If the object cannot be retrieved, the patient should be informed about the potential complications and escorted to a hospital for evaluation. Comprehensive diagnostic tests, such as chest and abdominal radiographs, should be performed to determine the status of the object and guide appropriate medical action, regardless of the patient's apparent condition. For radiolucent objects, computed tomography and diagnostic bronchoscopy are particularly useful in accurately locating the object.[94]

If the foreign body has entered the respiratory tract, before extracting the foreign object, its anatomic location (larynx, trachea, lobar, and segmental bronchi), shape, composition, and extent of entrapment by granulation tissue, inflammatory polyp, or edema must be identified to avoid the associated risks and further complications. Once localized, bronchoscopy is the treatment of choice for removal of aspirated items.[94]

If the foreign body has entered the gastrointestinal (GI) tract, its management depends on the patient's age, and the size, shape, composition, anatomic location of the object, and the time elapsed since ingestion. Impaction can occur at sites of physiologic angulation or pathologic narrowing, such as the pharynx, upper esophageal sphincter, middle third of the esophagus, lower esophageal sphincter, pylorus, duodenojejunal flexure, ileocecal junction, appendix, rectosigmoid junction, anus, or in patients with previous GI surgery or congenital gut malformations. The risk of aspiration, obstruction, or perforation determines the timing of intervention. Flexible endoscopy is the preferred procedure for retrieval of such objects from the GI tract.[94]

A foreign object should never remain in the esophagus for more than 24 hours to minimize the risk of serious complications. Once it passes into the stomach and beyond, the majority of foreign bodies—about 80–90%—pass uneventfully through the gastrointestinal tract and are expelled via the anus, including sharp or pointed objects, usually over a period of several days to weeks.[94]

Govila reported that endodontic instruments entering the gastrointestinal tract typically pass spontaneously in the feces within 4 days to 2 weeks. However, sharp objects carry a higher risk of perforation, so regular assessment and serial radiographic monitoring are recommended. While a high-bulk diet may be suggested to aid passage, there is no scientific evidence supporting the effectiveness of any specific diet in this regard.[99]

Sharp, pointed, or elongated objects longer than 6 cm typically fail to pass the proximal duodenum. Due to the high risk of perforation, urgent removal by endoscopy performed by a specialist is recommended before they reach the small intestine. Blunt or rounded objects wider than 2.5 cm are unlikely to pass the pylorus and generally require gastroscopic removal.[94]

Purgatives and laxatives should be avoided, as they increase peristaltic contractions and raise the risk of intestinal perforation. If the foreign object becomes impacted within mucosal folds, the ileocecal valve, or strictures, management may require rectoscopy, colonoscopy, or surgical intervention, depending on the object's location.[94]

Strategies to Prevent Aspiration/Ingestion in Dentistry

Prevention remains the most effective strategy to avoid aspiration or ingestion of foreign objects in dentistry. The use of a rubber dam is the simplest, most effective, and commonly recommended preventive measure for routine restorative and endodontic procedures. It not only reduces microbial contamination and the risk of swallowing or aspirating irrigants and instruments but also improves visibility, moisture control, and soft tissue retraction, thereby enhancing procedural efficacy. However, clamps themselves can pose a risk of aspiration or ingestion, so they should always be secured with dental floss.

Other protective measures include gauze throat screens, high-vacuum suction, customized impression trays, floss ligatures for small items, and adjusting the patient's position, especially for those with diminished protective reflexes. The gauze screen (4 × 4 inch) blocks small items from entering the oropharynx. For patients with strong gag reflexes, an upright chair position with the head turned to one side is recommended, and patients should be instructed to suppress swallowing if small items fall in the mouth.

All minor dental appliances, prostheses, and instruments should be secured with long floss for rapid retrieval if displaced. Cast restorations can also be prevented from aspiration by using dental floss. Finally, all instruments and materials should be carefully reviewed before, during, and after every procedure to minimize the risk of separation, aspiration, or ingestion.[94]

7.3 HYPOCHLORITE ACCIDENT

Sodium Hypochlorite Accidents

Sodium hypochlorite (NaOCl) is widely used as an endodontic irrigant due to its tissue-dissolving, antibacterial, and lubricating properties. However, it has an unpleasant odor, can damage clothing, and is more toxic than other irrigants. Its toxicity to vital tissues increases with concentration, so careful irrigation is essential to minimize tissue injury.[100]

Sodium hypochlorite (NaOCl) was first recognized for its antibacterial properties in 1843, when hand washing with hypochlorite between patients resulted in unusually low rates of infection transmission. It was first recorded as an endodontic irrigant in 1920 and is now routinely used worldwide.[101]

The ideal irrigant should

- Be an effective germicide and fungicide
- Be non-irritating to the periapical tissues
- Remain stable in solutions
- Have a prolonged antimicrobial effect

- Should be effective against the biofilms
- Have low surface tension
- Not interfere with repair of periapical tissues
- Be active in the presence of blood, serum
- Not stain tooth structure
- Be able to completely remove the smear layers, and be able to disinfect the underline dentine and its tubules [102]

Sodium Hypochlorite Properties

The chemical reactions verified between organic tissues and sodium hypochlorite are: [103]

1. Saponification reaction: sodium hypochlorite acts as organic and fat solvent degrading fatty acids, transforming them in to fatty acid salts (soap) and glycerol (alcohol), that reduces the surface tension of the remaining solutions.
2. Neutralization reaction: sodium hypochlorite neutralizes amino acids forming water and salt. With the exit of hydroxyl ions, there is reduction of pH. Hypochlorous acid, a substance presents in sodium hypochlorite, when in contact with the protein amino group, forms chloramines. Hypochlorous acid (HOCl-) and hypochlorite ions (OCl-) leads to amino acid degradation and hydrolysis.
3. Chloramination reaction: The chloramination reaction between chlorine and the amino group (NH) forms chloramines that interfere in cell metabolism. Chlorine (strong oxidant) presents antimicrobial action inhibiting bacterial enzymes leading to an irreversible oxidation of SH groups (sulphydryl group) of essential of bacterial enzymes.

Advantages of NaOCl

1. The powerful oxidative activity of hypochlorite not only dissolves the pulpal and dentinal tissues but also act as a potent antimicrobial agent. It is well recognized to be effective against a broad range of pathogens: gram-positive and gram-negative bacteria.
2. Effective concentration of NaOCl range from 2.6% or 5.25%. the dilution of Sodium hypochlorite (NaOCl) was suggested because it has been proved that concentration over 0.5% are cytotoxic.
3. Compared with chlorhexidine gel, Sodium hypochlorite (NaOCl) not only has a higher capacity to kill microorganisms but is also more able to remove cells from the root canal. Water is not effective in removing dentine debris from grooves in the apical portion of root canals.
4. The clinical efficacy Sodium hypochlorite (NaOCl) relates to its nonspecific ability to oxidize, hydrolyze and osmotically draw fluids out of tissues.[104]

Disadvantages of NaOCl

1. Acute inflammation followed by necrosis results when Sodium hypochlorite (NaOCl) comes in contact with vital tissues, causing severe inflammation and cellular destruction in all tissues except heavily keratinized epithelium.
2. The cytotoxic effect of 5.25% NaOCl on vital tissues results in hemolysis.
3. The severity of reaction depends on the concentration of the solution, its pH, and the duration of exposure. High concentrations can produce severe necrotic changes and irritation of the periodontal ligament.

4. Sodium hypochlorite (NaOCl) increases vascular permeability in blood vessels, likely due to tissue damage and release of chemical mediators such as histamine, causing immediate swelling and often profuse bleeding through the root canal when improperly used.
5. There is only one reported case of hypersensitivity to NaOCl, detectable via skin patch testing. Improper use can include inadvertent injection into the maxillary sinus or splashing into the eyes, with potential for facial nerve weakness and soft-tissue damage.
6. NaOCl has an unpleasant odor and can damage clothing on contact.
7. Two cases have been reported of NaOCl being inadvertently injected instead of an anesthetic solution: one causing severe palatal tissue necrosis, and the other causing edema in the pterygomandibular space and peritonsillar/pharyngeal areas, requiring ICU admission and intravenous opioids for pain.
8. In pediatric endodontics, careless use of NaOCl has caused damage to permanent tooth follicles, peripheral tissues, and oral mucosa.
9. A small number of cases report postoperative skin complications, long-term paresthesia, and altered nerve sensation following NaOCl use as an endodontic irrigant.

Predisposing Factors for Sodium Hypochlorite Accidents

1. Patient (Host)-Related Factors

- Gender: Females are more prone due to thinner bone density, making tissues more vulnerable to NaOCl extrusion injuries.
- Age: Young patients with open/wide apices and elderly patients with thin alveolar bone or root tips close to the sinus are at

higher risk. In elderly, compromised medical status and reduced body repair potential can worsen outcomes.

- Bone Quality: Less calcified alveolar bone and more marrow space (especially maxillary teeth) increases susceptibility.
- Medical Conditions: Immunocompromised patients, those with systemic diseases (e.g., diabetes, osteoporosis), and those undergoing certain therapies (like bisphosphonates) are more vulnerable.
- Anatomical Variations: Proximity to nerves and vasculature or facial venous variations increase danger of severe extrusions.[106,104]

2. Tooth-Related Factors

- Open/Wide Apex: Primary teeth, young permanent teeth, teeth with pathologic or physiologic resorption, immature apices, and non-vital teeth with apical lesions.
- Maxillary Teeth: Maxillary premolars and molars are more susceptible due to thin bone and proximity to the sinus.
- Perforations/Fenestrations: Apical perforations, lateral canals, and root fractures enhance risk for chemical escape.[105]
- Complex Anatomy: Multiple canals, accessory and lateral canals, sinus tracts, and bone fenestrations all increase risk.[106]

3. Operator-Related Factors

- Inexperience: Accidents are more common with less experienced clinicians (students, recent graduates, general practitioners).
- Technical Errors: Using piston-like actions with files, positive pressure irrigation with open-ended needles, large syringes, apical wedging of needles, and high force/pressure during irrigation promote extrusion.
- Inaccurate Working Length: Poor working length determination or apical canal preparation to a large size increases risk.[106]

4. NaOCl-Related Factors

- Irrigation Volume/Concentration: Using large amounts or high concentrations (above 3–5.25%) increases severity of injury.
- Solution Form: Buffered vs unbuffered NaOCl, and preheated solutions (questionable impact), duration and speed of irrigation, and longer tissue contact times may exacerbate accidents.[106]

Pathophysiology and Mechanisms

Sodium hypochlorite is a potent oxidizing agent. When extruded beyond the root apex or comes in contact with vital soft tissues, it causes:

- **Oxidation of proteins and lipids:** Leading to cell lysis, necrosis, and hemolysis.[96]
- **Chemical burns:** Causes localized/extrensive soft tissue necrosis and acute inflammatory responses, with both intraoral and extraoral swelling possible.
- **Vascular effects:** Increases vascular permeability, leading to rapid bleeding and edema. Sometimes causes ecchymosis or hematoma formation.[103]
- **Neurotoxicity:** Can damage nerves. Paraesthesia, anaesthesia, or even permanent nerve deficits (damage to the mental, infraorbital, and facial nerve branches) have been documented. Recovery is often slow—in some cases, months.[107]

How to Recognize a Hypochlorite Accident

1. Immediate severe pain (for 2-6 mins)
2. Ballooning/immediate edema in adjacent soft tissue because of perfusion to the loose connective tissue

3. Extension of edema to a larger site of face such as cheeks, periorbital region or lips
4. Ecchymosis on skin/mucosa as result of profuse interstitial bleeding
5. Profuse intraoral bleeding directly from root canal
6. Chlorine taste or smell because of injected NaOCl to maxillary sinus
7. Severe initial pain replaced with a constant discomfort or numbness, related to tissue destruction and distension
8. Reversible/persistent anesthesia
9. Possibility of secondary infection or spreading of former infection[107]

Rare Complications

- **Sinus involvement:** Accidental injection into the maxillary sinus leads to sinusitis, chlorine odor, and sometimes chronic consequences.[108]
- **Airway risk:** Large volume or concentration may cause severe swelling, risk airway obstruction and necessitating intensive care.[109]
- **Throat irritation or systemic toxicity:** Especially if large amounts swallowed (rare).
- **Bone necrosis:** Rare but documented in severe extrusion cases.

Management

Immediate Management

1. **Stop Procedure:** Immediately cease irrigation when pain, swelling, or bleeding is noticed.
2. **Irrigate Canal with Saline:** Flush the canal with copious saline to dilute and remove remaining NaOCl.

3. **Allow Bleeding:** If bleeding occurs, let it continue temporarily—it can help flush out the irritant from tissues.
4. **Pain Management:** Administer analgesics (ibuprofen, acetaminophen). For acute pain, local anaesthetic nerve block may be considered. [107,110]

Medical Management and Support Steroid Therapy: Prescribe systemic steroids (such as methylprednisolone or dexamethasone) for initial 2–3 days to control inflammation and minimize edema. Intravenous steroids may be warranted for severe cases.[99]

Antibiotics: Provide prophylactic antibiotics (suggested 7–10 days) to prevent secondary infection in cases with significant soft tissue involvement or immunocompromised patients.[99]

Cold Compresses: Apply ice packs over the affected area for the first 24hr (15-minute intervals) to limit swelling.

Warm Compresses: After 24hr, switch to gentle warm moist packs to encourage circulation and healing.

Saline Rinses: Advise gentle saline rinsing for approximately one week to maintain oral hygiene and support tissue repair.[107,110]

Monitoring and Communication Close Follow-Up: Daily review (in-person or telemedicine) to monitor for symptom progression, infection, or neurologic complications. Document all findings thoroughly.

Instruct and Reassure Patient: Provide clear verbal and written instructions regarding homecare, warning signs, and potential resolution time (weeks to months).

Hospital Referral: If swelling puts airway at risk, or for severe facial nerve deficits, immediately refer to hospital for specialist management and airway protection.[107,110]

Late Management (If needed)

- **Surgical Debridement:** For persistent necrosis or delayed healing, surgical intervention may be necessary.
- **Long-Term Rehabilitation:** Referral to oral medicine, surgery or neurology for prolonged paraesthesia, tissue loss, or nerve dysfunction. [107,110]

Documentation and Legal Considerations

- Record full details of the event, management steps, and correspondence with the patient for medico-legal records.[107]

Avoiding NaOCl accidents

The following steps can help clinicians avoid NaOCl accidents

1. Adequate access preparation
2. Good working length control
3. Irrigation needle placed 1mm to 3 mm short of working length
4. Needle placed passively and not locked in the canal
5. Irrigant expressed into the root canal slowly
6. Consistent in and out movements of the irrigating needle into canal space
7. "Flowback" of solution as it is expressed into the canal should be observed
8. Used side vented needles that are specifically designed for endodontic purposes.[106]

EMERGENCIES ASSOCIATED WITH LOCAL ANESTHESIA

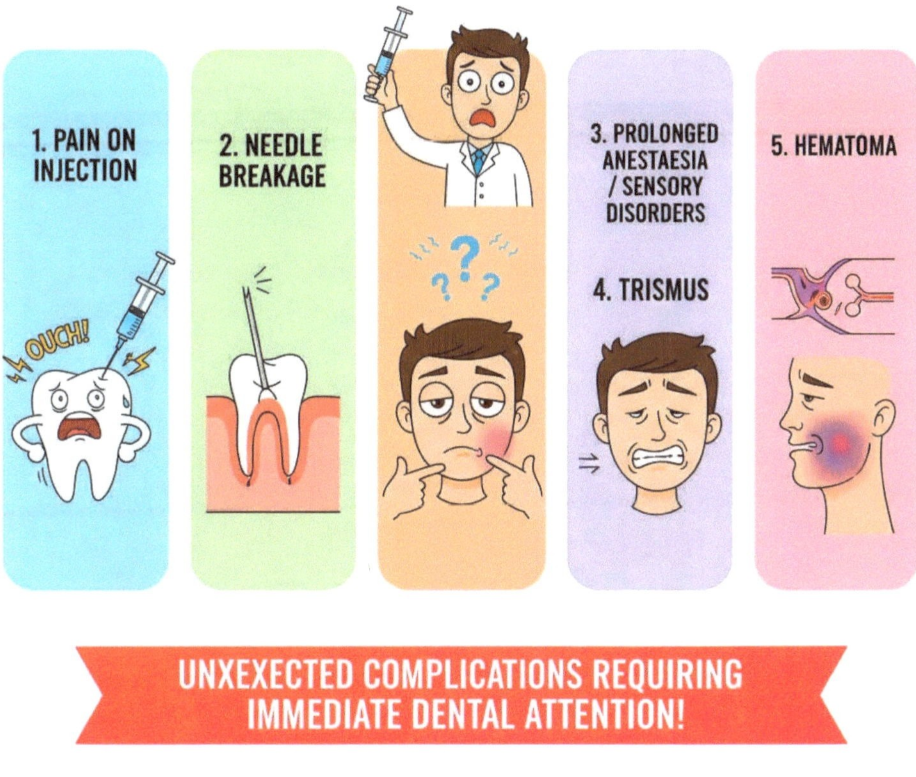

EMERGENCIES ASSOCIATED WITH LOCAL ANESTHESIA

8.1 PAIN ON INJECTION

Pain on injection can be due to specific circumstances such a temperate of the solution, velocity of injection, dull needles, needles with barbs, or aggressive insertion of the needle, damaging soft tissues, blood vessels, nerves, or the periosteum and causing more pain and other complications. The burning is dependent on the rate of injection and the acidity of the solution. Lidocaine causes an intense burning sensation when injected locally. When the needle penetrates a nerve, the patient may also feel a sudden "electric" shock, suddenly moving the head, with the risk of self-inflicted damage. In order to prevent discomfort, topical anesthetic application, warming anesthetics to body temperature, using a smaller-gauge needle (27 gauge), switching to a fresh needle when you have to inject multiple times in the same lesion or when you have multiple injection sites, and injecting slowly and with low pressure which reduces pain are done. A rate of 30 seconds per mL of solution is recommended. An inadequate injection site can lead to an intramuscular or intraneural injection blunting of the needle, side of injection anatomic structure (palate) it is unacceptable to feel a little pain during injection.[111]

8.2 NEEDLE BREAKAGE

Needle breakage in the oral cavity after local anesthesia is a rare complication, particularly since the introduction of non-reusable stainless steel dental needles. Most reported fractures involve 30-gauge needles and occur during inferior alveolar nerve blocks, typically due to incorrect injection technique, improper needle gauge selection, or unexpected patient movement. To prevent needle fracture, it is essential to check the injection needles beforehand, avoid using 30-gauge or short needles for inferior alveolar nerve blocks in adults or children (25–27 gauge is recommended), and ensure that needles are not bent during insertion into soft tissue.

If a needle breaks and is visible, it should be removed immediately using a hemostat. If the fragment is inaccessible, computed tomography (CT) should be performed to determine its location, and surgical removal under general anesthesia may be required. The literature generally recommends a superficial mucosal incision perpendicular to the needle trajectory followed by blunt supra-periosteal dissection to protect vital structures. Acham et al. (2018) analyzed 36 reports involving 59 needle breakage events and emphasized the importance of three-dimensional imaging to locate the fragment and assess surrounding structures such as blood vessels and the parotid gland. Their study found that 27 out of 57 cannula fragments were located in the pterygomandibular space, highlighting that the choice of removal technique, whether under general or local anesthesia, should be guided by the patient's systemic condition.[111]

8.3 PROLONGATION OF ANESTHESIA AND VARIOUS SENSORY DISORDERS

Prolonged anesthesia, paresthesia, or neuralgia can occur following dental local anesthetic blocks. These complications may be temporary, with sensation returning after days, weeks, or months, or in rare cases, permanent. They most commonly involve the lingual nerve (nervus lingualis), the inferior alveolar nerve (nervus mandibularis), or both. Nerve damage may result from direct trauma by the needle, disruption of intraneural blood supply causing hematoma, or trauma to the medial pterygoid muscle leading to trismus. Neurotoxicity of the anesthetic itself is also considered a possible mechanism, with procaine and tetracaine causing more damage compared to lidocaine or bupivacaine.

Although most cases of paresthesia or neuralgia are transient, permanent injury can occur if the anesthetic is injected directly into the nerve. Patients may experience secondary complications such as tongue biting, drooling, loss of taste, or speech difficulties due to prolonged numbness. Sullivan et al. conducted a randomized, double-blind, placebo-controlled trial on 496 patients with Bell's palsy and reported that initiating steroid treatment within three days of onset significantly improved the chances of full recovery at 3 and 9 months. Piccinni et al. found that the use of articaine or prilocaine is associated with a higher risk of paresthesia.

Management of nerve injury following dental local anesthesia should initially focus on pain control. Strategies to reduce the risk of anesthetic-related nerve injury include using a lower concentration of anesthetic for inferior alveolar nerve blocks (2% lidocaine is standard), avoiding repeated injections in the same site, and, when possible, using infiltration techniques with high-concentration agents like articaine instead of nerve blocks. Supplementation with low daily doses of vitamin B has also been recommended to support nerve healing and restore function.[111]

8.4 TRISMUS

Trismus is defined as a painful condition characterized by an inability to open the mouth normally. It can be caused by several factors, including multiple injections in a short period in the same area, intramuscular injections directly into the muscles, or trauma to muscles such as the lateral pterygoid or temporalis, which may result in hematoma formation and fibrosis. Other causes include needle fracture within muscles inserting into the styloid process, inaccurate needle positioning during inferior alveolar or posterior maxillary nerve blocks, inflammation of the masseter or other masticatory muscles, low-grade infections, and excessive volumes of local anesthetic solution in a confined space, which can lead to tissue expansion. In the acute phase, hemorrhage-induced pain causes muscle contraction, further limiting jaw movement. Some cases of trismus may resolve spontaneously; however, progression to chronic hypomobility or fibrous ankylosis can be prevented with early intervention. Recommended treatments include heat therapy, soft diet, prescription of analgesics, anti-inflammatory drugs, antibiotics (when infection is present), muscle relaxants, and physiotherapy. Typically, trismus resolves within six weeks, though the duration can range from four to twenty weeks. Prevention of trismus during local anesthesia requires awareness of anatomical landmarks and muscles. Palpation of the anterior ramus for the temporalis muscle and the pterygomandibular fold for the pterygoid muscle, along with appropriate needle angulation and bone contact, helps reduce the risk. For patients with limited mouth opening, anesthesia can be achieved using intraoral techniques such as the Vazirani-Akinosi closed-mouth mandibular nerve block or extraoral approaches.[112]

8.5 HEMATOMA

Hematoma formation is a recognized complication of local anesthesia, resulting from venous or arterial laceration. When an artery is punctured, the intra-arterial blood pressure can cause blood to effuse into surrounding soft tissues. High resistance during injection may serve as a warning of injecting against a blood vessel. The size and extent of a hematoma depend on the density and compactness of the affected tissue. Vein ruptures do not always result in a hematoma. Hematomas are often accompanied by discoloration or bruising of the area.

From an anatomical perspective, hematomas can occur in specific regions depending on the nerve block administered: anterior superior alveolar (infraorbital) nerve block may affect the area below the lower eyelid; incisive (mental) nerve block may affect the chin; buccal nerve blocks or palatal injections can cause intraoral hematomas; and posterior superior alveolar nerve blocks can result in extraoral hematomas in the lower buccal region of the mandible or intraorally distal to the maxillary tuberosity.

Prevention strategies include aspirating before injecting, using a short needle, and minimizing the number of needle penetrations. If swelling occurs immediately after injection, localized pressure should be applied for at least two minutes to control bleeding. Both swelling and discoloration typically resolve within 10 to 15 days. Ice packs should be applied during the first 24 hours, followed by intermittent hot moist packs and massage therapy using heparin cream. In cases of large hematomas, antibiotics may be prescribed to prevent secondary infection.[111]

POST-OPERATIVE ENDODONTIC EMERGENCIES

1. HIGH RESTORATION

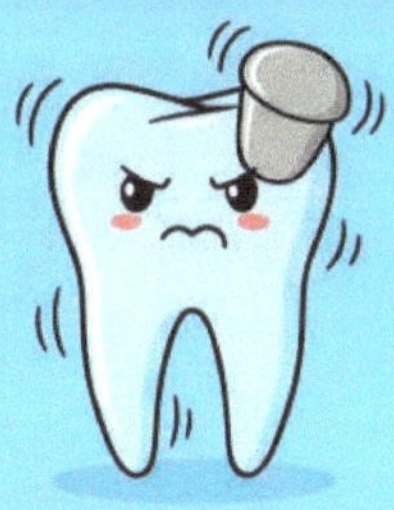

- New filling/crown feels 'high'
- Pain on biting or chewing
- Uneven bite

2. OVERFILLING

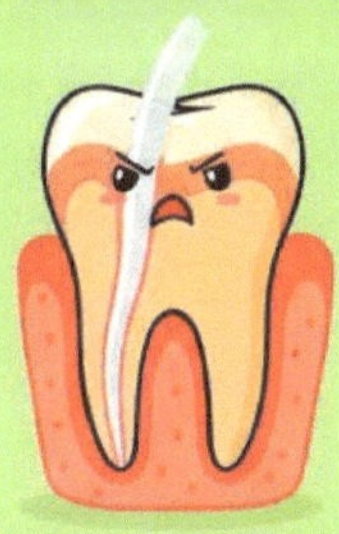

- Root canal filling material
- Pushes beyond the root tip
- Can cause inflammation & pain

3. ROOT FRACTURE

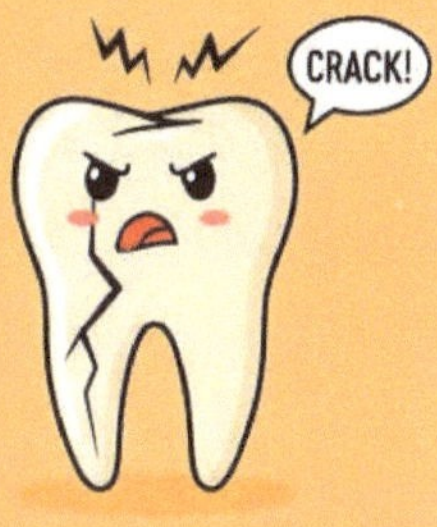

- Crack in the tooth root
- Often vertical
- Causes sharp pain with cheewing/temp changes

UNXEXECTED PAIN AFTER TREATMENT REQUIRES REQUIRES IMMEDIATE DENTAL ATTENTION!

POST-OPERATIVE ENDODONTIC MERGENCIES

Development of pain after endodontic intervention, commonly referred to as intra-appointment pain or flare-ups, represents one of the most frequent complications encountered in endodontics. The factors contributing to the sudden onset of such pain are complex and not fully understood. Most flare-ups arise from acute periradicular inflammation—manifesting as acute apical periodontitis or acute apical abscess—which occurs secondary to intracanal procedures. This acute inflammation can be triggered by any type of insult originating from the root canal system, whether mechanical, chemical, or microbial in nature.[113]

The following factors need to be considered in order to avoid the pain following sealing of the root canal system.

- **High restoration**
- **Overfilling**
- **Root fracture**

A number of hypothetical mechanisms that may be responsible for pain and/or swelling during endodontic therapy have been presented by many authors. These include chemical, mechanical or microbial injury to the periradicular tissue.[113]

Microbial Injury

A. Association with Specific Microorganisms

Most studies on endodontic flare-ups have focused on the association of clinical factors, while the role of specific microorganisms has received comparatively little attention. The environment within a root canal containing necrotic pulp tissue is highly conducive to the growth of diverse oral bacterial species, particularly strictly anaerobic bacteria with demanding nutritional requirements. Gomes et al. (1996) reported a significant association between Prevotella species and pain. Black-pigmented anaerobes, including Prevotella and Porphyromonas, were the most frequently recovered bacteria from cases presenting with tenderness to percussion. Moreover, the combined presence of Fusobacterium nucleatum, Prevotella, and Porphyromonas species is considered a risk factor for endodontic flare-ups, as these organisms can act synergistically to exacerbate periapical inflammatory lesions. Using the checkerboard DNA-DNA hybridization technique, Siqueira et al. (2001) identified Bacteroides forsythus, Porphyromonas gingivalis, Streptococcus constellatus, Prevotella intermedia, Fusobacterium nucleatum, and Fusobacterium periodonticum as the most prevalent species in cases diagnosed as acute apical abscess.[113]

B. Incomplete Bio-Mechanical Debridement of the Root Canal Space

Positive and negative interactions among members of the microbial community help maintain a relatively stable and balanced ecosystem within the root canal. Ideally, chemomechanical preparation should be completed in a single appointment to minimize disturbances to this balance. Incomplete chemomechanical preparation can disrupt the microbial equilibrium by eliminating some inhibitory species while leaving previously suppressed species to overgrow, potentially contributing to postoperative pain.

Situations in which incomplete biomechanical debridement may lead to postoperative pain include instrumentation that does not reach the apical constriction, undetected or missed canals, and anatomical complexities of the root canal system such as C-shaped canals, apical deltas, multiple foramina, and furcation accessory canals.[113]

C. Secondary Intra-Radicular Infection

Secondary intraradicular infections occur when microorganisms gain access to the root canal system during treatment, between appointments, or even after the completion of endodontic therapy. Such infections typically arise following a breach in the aseptic chain. The main sources of recontamination during treatment include remnants of dental plaque, calculus, or caries on the tooth crown, as well as a leaking or improperly placed rubber dam. Microorganisms can also infiltrate the root canal system between appointments if there is leakage or loss of the temporary restoration.[113]

D. Increase of the Oxidation-Reduction Potential

It has been theorized that changes in the oxidation–reduction potential (Eh) within the root canal environment may contribute to exacerbations following endodontic procedures. The introduction of oxygen into the root canal during treatment could promote the overgrowth of facultative bacteria that survived chemo-mechanical debridement. This theory is supported by microbial isolates from teeth experiencing acute exacerbations during endodontic therapy, where the recovered microorganisms were predominantly aerobic and facultative, mainly facultative streptococci, with no obligate anaerobes detected.[113]

Mechanical Injury

Instrumentation beyond the apical foramen is a recognized iatrogenic factor contributing to post-operative endodontic pain. Typically, a distance of 0.5 to 2 mm short of the radiographic apex is considered acceptable for root canal instrumentation. However, due to factors such as X-ray angulations, deviations of the apical foramen, or superimposed anatomical structures, a canal appearing to terminate 0.5–2 mm from the radiographic apex may actually extend into the periradicular tissues. Consequently, a working length that radiographically ends 0–2 mm short of the apex does not guarantee avoidance of over-instrumentation. To enhance accuracy, radiographic measurements of working length should be supplemented with electronic apex locator determinations. Iatrogenic over-instrumentation can enlarge the apical foramen, allowing increased influx of exudates and blood into the root canal, which in turn may enhance the nutrient supply for residual bacteria.[113]

Chemical Injury

Irrigation solutions and intracanal medicaments are primarily used within the root canal to aid in cleaning and disinfecting the dentinal walls. However, these substances often come into contact with periapical tissues, either through accidental extrusion beyond the apex or via leaching. Sodium hypochlorite (NaOCl) is the most widely used endodontic irrigant due to its strong antimicrobial properties and ability to dissolve pulp tissue. While NaOCl at low concentrations (0.5%) is generally nontoxic and rapidly neutralized by circulating blood, higher concentrations are highly cytotoxic and can cause severe tissue irritation upon contact. Most complications associated with NaOCl arise from accidental extrusion beyond the apical foramen, known as a "sodium hypochlorite accident." Such accidents can trigger immediate, severe pain, rapidly increasing swelling, hemorrhage through the tooth, interstitial bleeding with ecchymosis of surrounding tissues, and, in some cases, secondary infection or paresthesia. Accidental extrusion typically occurs when excessive pressure is applied during irrigation or if the needle tip becomes bound in the canal, preventing coronal flow of the solution. Given its potent tissue-dissolving capacity, NaOCl in contact with periapical tissues can rapidly induce necrosis.[113]

Incidence

The reported incidence of postoperative endodontic pain varies widely, ranging from 1.7% to 70%. Although most studies are either randomized controlled trials or prospective studies, direct comparison between them is challenging due to differences in study design, the preoperative condition of the treated teeth, treatment procedures or techniques, timing of pain assessment, the scales used for pain measurement, and the severity thresholds included in the statistical analysis. These variations are summarized in Tables 1 and 2 below.[114]

Table 9.1 Reported incidence of Postoperative Pain (all intensities) by different studies

Author/yr.	Teeth	Incidence (%)	Related factor(s)
Albashaheir (1998)	291	38% multi-visits; 27% single visit	Non-vital pulps
Aqrabawi (2006)	146	8 h: 74%; 1 d: 69%; 2 d: 46%	Hand and rotary instrumentation technique has no diff.
Almeida (2012)	126	3% moderate; 19% mild	No diff. between NaOCl and chlorhexidine irrigation
Byram (2009)	306	69.9% single visit; 69.2% in two visits; 4.6% severe	No diff. between vital and non-vital; no diff. b/n single and multiple visits
Ehrmann (2003)	223	4 h: 37%; 1 d: 23%; 2 d: 38%	Ledermix found to be effective in pain control
El Mubarak (2010)	234	12 h: 9%	Preoperative pain
Fava (1998)	60	2 days: 2%	No diff. between Ca(OH)2 and steroid-antibiotic dressing
Gesi (2006)	256	7 days: 10%	Associated with overfilling
Glennon (2004)	272	64.7% (<10% severe)	Presence of preoperative pain, tooth type, systemic steroid, preoperative swelling
Gotler (2012)	274	63.8% vital; 38.5% necrotic; 48% retreatment	Vital pulps induce more pain
Henry (2001)	41	1 d: 56%; 2 d: 33%; 3 d: 27%	Symptomatic necrotic teeth
Polycarpou (2005)	175	12%	Presence of preoperative pain; female gender
Risso (2008)	121	10.5% single visit; 23% two visit	Presence of pre-operative pain

Siqueira (2002)	627	Mild pain: 10%; Moderate: 3.3%; Severe: 1.9%	Previously symptomatic teeth without periradicular lesions
Segura-Egea (2009)	176	37% anterior; 56% posterior	Mandibular > max.; Irreversible pulpitis and acute apical periodontitis
Sadaf (2014)	140	42.9%	Preoperative pain, female gender
Najma (2014)	474	2.53%	Mandibular teeth
Mor (1992)	334	4.2%	Higher in non-vital teeth without apical radiolucency
Torabinejad (1994)	588	6%	Preoperative pain, apprehension, intracanal medication
Ng (2004)	415	40.2%, less than 12% severe	Female, molars, size of periradicular lesion smaller 3mm, single visit
Walton (1993)	80	70% all intensities; low severe	No diff. between administration of antibiotic or non administration

Related Factors

1. **Number of Visits:** Considerable controversy exists regarding whether endodontic therapy should be completed in a single appointment or multiple visits. Many practitioners favour a two-visit approach to allow for a symptom-free period after canal debridement before obturation. Factors often cited in this debate include the risk of coronal filling leakage, potential reinfection from periapical or periodontal pathogens, incomplete elimination of intracanal or intratubular bacteria, and the relative ease of managing any subsequent infections.[114]

2. **Retreatment**: Incomplete or inadequate root canal treatment has been suggested as a contributing factor in post-treatment complications. Torabinejad and Imura reported a higher incidence of inter-appointment emergencies following endodontic retreatment compared to initial root canal treatment. [114]
3. **Presence of Pre-operative Pain:** The presence and severity of pre-operative pain appear to strongly influence the development of post-operative pain following initial root canal preparation. This can be explained by the fact that virulent clonal types of pathogenic bacterial species present in the root canal system are responsible for the pre-operative symptoms. Extrusion of these virulent microorganisms into the periradicular tissues during instrumentation has a greater potential to induce or exacerbate periradicular inflammation compared to non-virulent microorganisms that did not cause pre-operative symptoms.[114]

Table 9.2 Different studies reported incidence of sever postoperative pain – flare ups- with any related factors

Author/yr.	Teeth	Incidence (%)	Related factor (s)
Walton (1992)	946 visits	3.7% flare up	Pulpal necrosis with painful apical pathosis
Alacam (2002)	474	7.17%	More in mandibular
Iqbal (2009)	6580	0.39 %	Presence of a periapical lesion
Al Negrish (2006)	120	2days:11.6% 7days: 3.6%	No. of visits has no effect
Alves Vde (2010)	408	1.71%	Presence of periradicular radiolucency

Author/yr.	Teeth	Incidence (%)	Related factor (s)
Oginni (2004)	227	8.1% in multiple visits, 18.3% single visit	Preoperative pain
Eleazer (1998)	402	8% two visits; 3% one visit	Advantage of single visit
Syed (2012)	1328	12h:9%; 24h:8.6%	Old, female, preoperative pain
Udoye (2011)	175	10%	No factors

4. **Pulp & Periradicular Condition:** Necrotic pulps create an environment conducive to the growth of diverse oral bacterial species, particularly strictly anaerobic bacteria. Since microorganisms are the primary causative agents of acute periradicular inflammation—whether it occurs pre-operatively or post-operatively—it is theoretically reasonable to suggest that post-operative pain is more likely to occur following instrumentation of necrotic pulps compared to vital pulps. Most studies have found a positive correlation between pulpally necrotic teeth with painful apical pathosis and an increased incidence of flare-ups.[114]

5. **Intra-canal Medicaments:** Siquiera et al. (2002) stated that the intra-canal procedures based on the maximum elimination of the irritant including antimicrobial intra-canal dressing are valuable tool to control endodontic infections and theoretically prevent postoperative pain.
   - **Calcium Hydroxide [Ca $(OH)_2$** Ca $(OH)_2$ has been found to be quickly and highly effective against some microorganisms related to severe clinical symptoms. Despite the proven antimicrobial activity of Ca $(OH)_2$, many studies showed

its limited effect on post-treatment pain after the chemo-mechanical root canal preparation.

- **Steroids** According to the findings of the clinical studies performed to correlate the steroid intracanal medicaments and postoperative pain, there is no clear direct preventive effect of these medicaments to endodontic flare-ups. They may have an anti-inflammatory effect but this reduction in inflammation only shows some effect in reducing the severity of this pain after some hours.[114]

Table 9.3 Different studies investigated the relationship between intra-canal medicaments and postoperative endodontic pain

Author	Teeth/ diagnosis	Medicament tested	Finding
Siqueira (2002)	627/ necrotic pulps	$Ca(OH)_2$ / para-monochlorophenol paste	Low incidence of flare-ups after dressing with $Ca(OH)_2$ /camphorated para-monochlorophenol paste.
Ehrmann (2003)	Necrotic with acute apical periodontitis	$Ca(OH)_2$; Ledermix; placebo	Ledermix is an effective intracanal medicament for the control of postoperative pain.
Richard (2003)	140	$Ca(OH)_2$ intracanal dressing	Unrelated to the incidence and/or severity of post treatment pain
Anjaneyulu (2014)	Review	$Ca(OH)_2$	No clear evidence of its effect on post-treatment pain
Trope (1990)		$Ca(OH)_2$; Ledermix; placebo	No significant difference among the three intracanal medicaments.

Author	Teeth/ diagnosis	Medicament tested	Finding
Menakaya (2015)		Mixture of saline/ $Ca(OH)_2$ vs. chlorhexidine paste	Postoperative pain was lower in the normal saline/$Ca(OH)_2$ treatment group
Moskow A. (1984)	50	Dexamethasone solution	Significant reduction of pain at 24 h.
Negm (2001)	988	Corticosteroid antibiotic combination	Complete relief of pain after 24 h. (pain reduction)
Rimmer (1991)	Non vital teeth	$Ca(OH)_2$, Ledermix, formocresol intra-canal med.	Lower flare-up scores with steroid/antibiotic mixtures
Fava (1998)	60 incisors with acute apical periodontitis	$Ca(OH)_2$, steroid antibiotic combination	No difference in pain incidence and severity between the two intracanal medicaments.
Walton (2003)	140	$Ca(OH)_2$ vs. sterile cotton pellet	$Ca(OH)_2$ was unrelated to the incidence and/ or severity of post treatment pain.
Singh (2013)	64 teeth, necrotic pulps and acute apical periodontitis	$Ca(OH)_2$ paste with chlorhexidine gel; 2% chlorhexidine gel; $Ca(OH)_2$	Chlorhexidine alone and $Ca(OH)_2$ plus chlorhexidine gave rise to less pain than calcium hydroxide alone or no dressing at all.

6. **Irrigating Solutions:** The type of irrigating solution used makes little difference in the incidence of post-operative discomfort, providing that the irrigating solution is not forced beyond the foramen of the tooth. Since the induction of pain in endodontic therapy is multi factorial, it is difficult to attribute a lower pain incidence specifically to the use of any particular irrigant. Bashety K (2010) reported more pain in teeth irrigated using 5.25% sodium hypochlorite when compared to the pain in teeth irrigated using 2% chlorhexidine solution. In contrast, Almeida et al. (2012) found no difference between post operative pain in teeth irrigated with NaOCl or chlorohexidine solutions. [114]

7. **Systemic Medication**
   - **Systemic Steroids:** The use of systemic steroids for the prevention of post-operative endodontic pain has been investigated with varying results. In addition to oral administration, local injections around the treated tooth—such as intraligamental or supraperiosteal injections—have also been studied. In his 2002 review, Marshal JG reported that systemic steroids are effective as an adjunct, but not a replacement, for proper endodontic treatment in reducing post-treatment pain. Steroids are particularly beneficial for patients presenting with moderate to severe pain and a clinical diagnosis of pulpal necrosis associated with periapical radiolucency.
   - **Systemic Antibiotics Prophylaxis:** Since bacterial infection of the periradicular tissues is the major causative factor in endodontic flare-ups, it has been proposed that prophylactic antibiotics might prevent such complications. However, the routine use of antibiotics in healthy patients for this purpose

remains controversial, as overprescription can contribute to bacterial resistance and patient sensitization. Evidence from controlled clinical trials provides little to no support for the idea that antibiotics reduce post-operative pain.[114]

Table 9.4 Different studies investigated the effect of systemic steroids on post-operative endodontic pain

Author	Systemic steroid/dose	Finding
Marshal (2002)	4 mg of dexamethasone intramuscular	Significantly reduced both the incidence and severity of pain after 4 hours after single-visit endodontic therapy
Krasner (1986)	0.75 mg dexamethasone or placebo orally	Administrations of oral dexamethasone significantly reduced post-operative pain after 8 and 24 hours
Elieazer (1994)	methylprednisolone intra-ligamentally	Significantly reduced the frequency and intensity of postoperative pain
Mehrvarzfar (2008)	Supraperiosteal injection of dexamethasone	Could be effective in reduction or prevention of postoperative pain during the first 24 h.
Jalalzadeh (2010)	Prednisolone orally (30 mg) before RCT; placebo	Reduced postendodontic pain.

Table 9.5 Administration of different prophylactic antibiotics on post-operative endodontic pain

Author	Teeth	Antibiotic	Finding
Henry (2001)	Symptomatic necrotic teeth	Penicillin 500 mg capsules for 7 days	Did not reduce pain, percussion pain, swelling.
Walton (1993)		Prophylactic penicillin	No difference between administration or non-administration of antibiotics after 48 h.
Fouad (1996)	Pulp necrosis; apical periodontitis	Penicillin and placebo	No difference was found between the groups of administration and non-administration of penicillin.
Pickenpaugh (2001)	Symptomatic necrotic teeth	3 mg prophylactic amoxicillin	No effect on the endodontic flare-up.
Torabinejad (1994)		Erythromycin; Methylprednisolone plus penicillin	All are more effective than placebo within the first 48 h following RCT.

Author	Teeth	Antibiotic	Finding
Morse (1990)	Necrotic pulp / chronic apical periodontitis	Single dose – long acting 1 gm tablet of cephalosporin	Prophylactic administration of antibiotics significantly reduced the incidence of flare-ups.
Abbott (1988)	Pulpal necrosis / peri-apical pathosis	Penicillin and erythromycin	Low incidence of flare-ups, with no difference between penicillin or erythromycin.
Alsomadi (2015)		Ibuprofen 400 mg before; same regimen + amoxicillin	Antibiotic prescription could result in less post-endodontic pain.

- **Non-Steroidal Anti-Inflammatory Drugs (NSAIDs)** Non-steroidal anti-inflammatory drugs (NSAIDs) are increasingly used primarily for their analgesic effect rather than as anti-inflammatory agents. Since periapical inflammation is a major contributor to post-treatment pain, NSAIDs may be effective in managing this discomfort. Administration of analgesics either before or after treatment has been shown to significantly reduce the incidence and severity of endodontic flare-ups.[114]

Table 9.6 Different studies investigate systemic prophylaxis of NSAIDs on post-operative pain

Author	NSAID	Finding
Walton and Fouad (1991)	—	Analgesics and antiinflammatory drugs were found to have a significantly higher incidence of flareups.
Torabinejad (1994)	Ibuprofen	More effective than placebo in controlling pain.
Menhinick (2004)	600 mg ibuprofen and 1000 mg acetaminophen	More effective than ibuprofen alone for the management of postoperative endodontic pain.
Monke (2000)	Prophylactic etodolac; ibuprofen; placebo	Ibuprofen was more effective in pain reduction than etodolac and placebo.
Gopikrishnan (2003)	Rofecoxib, ibuprofen, or placebo (prophylactically)	Both rofecoxib and ibuprofen provided better pain relief than placebo at 4 and 8 hours.
Nekofar (2003)	Meloxicam; piroxicam; placebo	No significant differences between the three groups.
Attar (2008)	Ibuprofen before RCT	Did not reduce postoperative pain.

Author	NSAID	Finding
Negm (1989)	Piroxicam and diclofenac	Piroxicam and diclofenac were superior to placebo in controlling postoperative pain.
Metri (2016)	Diclofenac 30 minutes before RCT	Postendodontic pain was substantially reduced.
Mokhtari (2016)	Indomethacin 25 mg or ibuprofen 400 mg	Both ibuprofen and indomethacin significantly reduced postoperative pain.

Technique of Instrumentation

All instrumentation techniques are reported to cause apical extrusion of debris, even when preparation is maintained short of the apical foramen. The difference lies in the extent of debris extrusion, as some techniques tend to extrude more than others. Crown-down techniques using rotary instruments combined with abundant irrigation theoretically have the potential to reduce the risk of flare-ups. Mechanical preparation with rotary instruments has been associated with less post-operative pain compared to hand instrumentation; however, Aqrabawi et al. reported no statistically significant difference in post-treatment pain between teeth prepared with manual or NiTi rotary techniques.

Creating a glide path prior to canal instrumentation can reduce the amount of apically extruded debris in curved canals. The use of a patency file during all stages of canal preparation may improve debris removal from the apical portion of the root canal, maintaining canal patency. This facilitates drainage of inflammatory exudates, decompresses periapical tissues, allows oxygen to enter (which is lethal for anaerobic bacteria), and enables better contact of intracanal dressings with living periapical tissues. Regarding working length determination, Kara (2014) found no difference in postoperative pain between measurements obtained using an electronic apex locator versus digital radiography.[114]

Psychological Factors

Fear of dentists and dental procedures, along with anxiety, apprehension, and other psychological factors, can significantly influence a patient's perception of pain and their reaction threshold. Torabinejad and colleagues observed an association between preoperative apprehension and the occurrence of post-operative pain, suggesting that patients who are more anxious or fearful before endodontic treatment may experience greater discomfort following the procedure.[114]

Gender, Age, Tooth Location and Type

Fear of dentists, anxiety, apprehension, and related psychological factors can strongly affect a patient's pain perception and response threshold. Torabinejad and colleagues reported that preoperative apprehension is associated with an increased likelihood of post-operative pain, indicating that patients who are anxious or fearful prior to endodontic treatment may experience more intense discomfort afterward.[114]

Prevention

Clinical procedures: Although there is no specific clinical procedure or medication found to prevent endodontic post-operative pain, some clinical tips need to be followed in an effort to minimize its occurrence.

- Maintaining the aseptic condition during intracanal procedures: Asepsis is paramount in endodontic therapy to prevent infection in vital cases or introduction of new microbial species in cases of infected necrotic pulps. Thus, clinicians should be aware of the need to perform endodontic treatment under strictly aseptic conditions as some cases of secondary infections may even be more difficult to treat than primary infections and may cause flare-ups, persistent symptoms and /or failure of the root canal treatment.
- Selection of instrumentation techniques that extrude less amounts of debris apically.
- Completion of the biomechanical debridement of the root canal space in the first visit: Maximum removal of irritants from the root canal system may reduce the risks of inter-appointment discomfort caused by the remaining virulent microorganisms.
- Use of an anti-inflammatory or anti-microbial intracanal medicament between appointments in the treatment of infected cases.
- Instrumentation to 1-2 mm shorter than the radiographical apex and confirming the working length by electronic apex locators, in cases of infected canals exhibiting periapical involvement and pre-treatment symptoms, where the possibility of developing flare-ups is high, the clinician should take maximum care to confine the instrumentation short of the radiographic apex avoiding extrusion of debris from the canal into the periradicular tissues.
- Psychological preparation of patients: (particularly those with preoperative pain) will decrease inter-appointment symptoms in the mild to moderate levels.

- Avoidance leaving the root canal open for the purpose of drainage. Leaving the tooth open is the most direct way to permit the re-infection of the root canal system in addition to overcome any previous attempts to eradicate microorganisms within root canal system.
- To minimize NaOCl accidents, the irrigating needle should be placed short of the working length, fit loosely in the canal and the solution must be injected using a gentle flow rate. Constantly moving the needle up and down during irrigation prevents wedging of the needle in the canal and provides better irrigation. The use of irrigation tips with side venting reduces the possibility of forcing solutions into the periapical tissues.

The reported incidence of post-operative endodontic pain varies widely, though severe pain or flare-ups occur relatively infrequently. The primary etiology is microbial injury to the periapical tissues, often resulting from the extrusion of infected debris during canal instrumentation. Currently, there is no definitive evidence that any specific technique, intracanal agent, or systemic medication can reliably prevent this complication. Some local or systemic medications may help manage the pain once it occurs, but they do not act as preventive measures. Nevertheless, clinicians should be encouraged to follow evidence-based guidelines and adopt procedural strategies that have the potential to reduce the risk and severity of post-operative endodontic pain.[114]

9.1 OVERFILLING / OVEREXTENDED OBTURATION

Overfilled root canals commonly occur due to factors such as inflammatory apical root resorption, incompletely formed root apex, inaccurate working length determination, or instrumentation beyond the apical foramen. In these situations, overfilling happens because achieving an apical stop is difficult. Consequently, the success rate in such cases drops to around 76%, compared to the general 75–95% success reported for routine root canal treatment. Treatment failures following overfilling with gutta-percha (GP) are usually attributed to persistent root canal infection, reinfection from apical transportation of bacteria during over-instrumentation, or a foreign body reaction to the overextended GP. Management of root canal failure due to GP overfilling can involve nonsurgical retreatment, periradicular surgery, or a combination of both.

Periradicular surgery is typically indicated in cases of significant overextension of filling material associated with periradicular pathosis, true periradicular cysts with fully enclosed epithelium-lined cavities that are unlikely to resolve with nonsurgical treatment, persistent periradicular lesions, or to correct deficiencies in previous treatment. However, in younger patients, periradicular surgery is often less satisfactory due to potential discomfort, the need for patient cooperation, and the possibility of behavior management challenges during future dental appointments.[115,116]

The periradicular cyst observed in this case can be attributed to over-instrumentation during the previous root canal treatment, which caused trauma to the periapical tissues, apical transportation of intracanal bacteria, lack of an adequate apical seal, and overfilling with gutta-percha (GP). These factors likely evoked persistent chronic inflammation with epithelial proliferation, ultimately leading to cyst formation. Despite the patient's young age, periapical surgery was chosen because the endodontic failure involved a sizable periradicular cyst, over-instrumented apical portion, and dense overfilled GP.

Nonsurgical retreatment, such as removal of GP using Hedstrom files and solvents like chloroform or xylene, may only be effective in cases of poorly condensed fillings. In overextended obturations with well-adapted GP, fragments often remain in the periapical tissues, limiting the success of nonsurgical approaches. Furthermore, failed root canal cases with periradicular cysts caused by apical transportation or procedural errors are generally better managed surgically due to the complex canal anatomy and the low predictability of achieving complete debridement nonsurgically.

Since inadequate apical sealing and microbial contamination are primary contributors to periapical lesions, achieving a proper apical seal with a root-end material of superior sealing ability is critical. In this case, mineral trioxide aggregate (MTA) was selected for root capping due to its biocompatibility, capacity to stimulate osteogenesis and cementogenesis, antibacterial activity, excellent marginal adaptation, and dimensional stability. MTA's hydrophilicity, radiopacity, and ability to set in the presence of blood further supported its use.

Root capping with MTA preserved the root length and crown-to-root ratio while avoiding root-end procedures that could compromise a thinned or weakened apical portion. At six months, partial dislodgement of MTA into the regenerated bone was observed, likely due to pressure from bone remodeling during periapical healing. This phenomenon, also reported in other cases of apically extruded MTA, suggests that periapical tissues possess an intrinsic capacity to restore their original structure, potentially displacing foreign material in the process. The absence of retention for the MTA capping may have contributed to its partial displacement, representing a potential limitation of root capping versus traditional root-end filling procedures. Despite this drawback, MTA root capping can offer clinical advantages in selected cases, as it ensures an effective apical seal and promotes periapical healing. Future use of materials that bond to the root surface while retaining MTA's biological and sealing properties may further enhance outcomes in similar cases.[115,116]

9.2 POST FRACTURE / ROOT FRACTURE

According to the American Association of Endodontists, a vertical root fracture (VRF) is defined as a longitudinal fracture of the root that originates at the apex and propagates toward the coronal portion of the tooth. Literature reports indicate that VRF is the third most common cause of extraction in endodontically treated teeth. This condition poses a significant threat to the long-term prognosis of the affected tooth during and after root canal treatment. Diagnosing vertical root fractures can be challenging, as definitive identification is often difficult and may rely on predictive assessment rather than direct confirmation. Clinically, the presentation of VRF may mimic other conditions, such as periodontal disease or failed root canal treatment, making differential diagnosis essential. Radiographic detection of VRFs is also problematic because classical radiographic signs are not consistently present in every case. The accuracy of radiographic diagnosis depends on multiple factors, including correct angulation, appropriate contrast and density settings, and the clinician's expertise in interpreting subtle radiographic features.[117,118]

Histopathogenesis of Vertical Root Fractures

Vertical root fractures create a pathway for various irritants—such as bacteria and their metabolites, necrotic pulpal tissue, sealer components, and food debris—to enter the fracture site during mastication. The bacterial contamination can originate either from the gingival sulcus or from the root canal itself, particularly if the canal has not been completely disinfected. This infiltration of irritants contributes to periodontal breakdown, often resulting in deep probing defects that are characteristic of vertical root fractures. Although the "hollow tube theory" remains controversial, the fracture nonetheless exposes a significant area of the canal space, allowing substances to enter, degrade, and act as persistent irritants to the surrounding tissues.[117,118]

Incidence and distribution according to the type of tooth in Vertical root fractures Premolars are the most susceptible teeth for vertical root fracture followed by molars, incisors and cuspids in descending order.

The most susceptible roots to fracture are maxillary and mandibular premolars, mesial roots of mandibular molars and mandibular incisors.

Root depressions in the mesial roots of mandibular molars and buccal roots of bifurcated maxillary premolars are the anatomical entities that can predispose the roots to fracture. Gher et al. suggested a low incidence of 2.3% of vertical root fractures among teeth. Patterns of vertical root fracture in vital and endodontically treated teeth Grippo suggested that mechanical loading factors affecting teeth are magnitude, frequency, locations and direction of force. In vital teeth, excessive masticatory force leads to the attrition of occlusal surface. Forces concentrated at weaker apical part, initiate crack, which progresses coronally. In roots weakened due to endodontic treatment or post, crack begins at the apex or mid root or some other positions. Predisposing factors for vertical root fractures in non-vital teeth Root canal anatomy Roots narrower in mesiodistal dimension and with developmental depression such as mesial root of mandibular molars and buccal roots of premolars are more susceptible to fracture. Reduced curvature radius of roots in buccal and lingual areas. Ratio of canal width to the width of total root also increases the risk of root fracture. Change in dentin characteristics in endodontically treated teeth Dentin of pulpless teeth exhibits more plastic deformation than does that of normal teeth. Dehydration of human dentin increases its Young's modulus, in other words it increases stiffness, which is attributed to the change in collagen cross linking of root dentin in endodontically treated teeth. Residual dentin thickness after removal of intracanal procedures [117,118]

- Excessive removal of dentin during coronal enlargement of canal and post space preparation.
- Round canal preparation in an oval canal. This decreases the remaining dentin thickness and increases the susceptibility to fracture.
- Long term calcium hydroxide as a root canal dressing may increase the risk of root fracture. Calcium hydroxide causes change in the organic matrix, which is due to disruption of link between the hydroxyapatite crystals and collagenous network in dentin. Root fractures associated with corrosion products of pins and posts also contribute to root fractures. In a study out of 468 teeth with root fractures, evidence of a fracture could be demonstrated radiographically by the presence of corrosion products from the pin or post or by dissolution of the pin in 71.8% of the cases. Use of spreader and vertical root fracture The wedging effect of a spreader during lateral condensation of root canal obturation can induce vertical root fracture (VRF). To reduce this risk, it is recommended to prepare canals with increased taper, which allows for a more uniform distribution of stresses during lateral condensation.

Obturation techniques and VRF: Excessive forces applied during lateral condensation are known to produce apical strain, contributing to VRFs. In contrast, obturation techniques such as Obtura and Thermafil generate more coronal strain and can cause thermal expansion of the root dentin, which may also influence fracture risk.

Post placement and VRF: Tapered end posts can create a wedging effect near the apex, which is particularly severe for smaller diameter posts with shallow embedment. Parallel-sided posts distribute stress more evenly, while larger diameter posts placed deeper within the canal provide the most favorable stress distribution. Rigid posts, such as zirconia, are more likely to induce vertical root fractures.

Studies examining fracture susceptibility in endodontically treated teeth over five years—including teeth with or without posts and with full or partial coverage restorations—found that all 220 teeth survived during the study period. These findings suggest the need for further research to clarify the protective role of posts and restorations in preventing VRFs.

In vital teeth, small cracks, tooth infractions, or acute trauma to anterior teeth from heavy masticatory loads or biting on hard objects may act as precursors for VRFs. Another significant factor is the cracked tooth syndrome, which can predispose vital teeth to fracture.

In non-endodontically treated teeth, VRFs have been reported as relatively common in certain populations. For instance, a study in a Chinese cohort found a predilection for males, with all 64 affected teeth being molars with minimal or no restorations. Severe attrition due to dietary habits was implicated as the primary cause of fractures in this population.

Overall, VRFs are influenced by a combination of anatomical, mechanical, and iatrogenic factors, including obturation technique, post design, and preexisting structural defects.[117,118]

Recommendations in Cases of Vertically Fractured Teeth

1. CBCT can be valuable in the diagnosis and treatment of vertical root fracture, after the routine clinical and radiographic examination.
2. It is essential to determine the necessity of a post in endodontically treated teeth
   - For maxillary incisors with only access cavities no posts are required.
   - For posterior teeth with sufficient tooth structure remaining after tooth preparation, posts are not required.
   - A post and core may help prevent coronal fractures, when the remaining coronal tooth structure is very thin after tooth preparation.
   - Among the posts, threaded posts cause highest strain and incidence of root fracture. Parallel sided, serrated posts cause highest success rate.

Posts when indicated should be passive, and use of fiber reinforced composite posts should be considered whenever possible.

- Complete coverage restorations are necessary in case of endodontically treated posterior teeth except when the destruction is limited only to access cavity.
- More flexible and less tapered finger spreaders are safer than stiff, conventional hand spreader.
- Root strength can be improved by removing the smear layer in case of fiber posts.
- Resin based sealers like AH-26 can be used to strengthen root canal.

Over flared root canals which are more susceptible to vertical root fracture can be reinforced by MTA rather than gutta-percha, resilon or composite.[117,118]

CONCLUSION

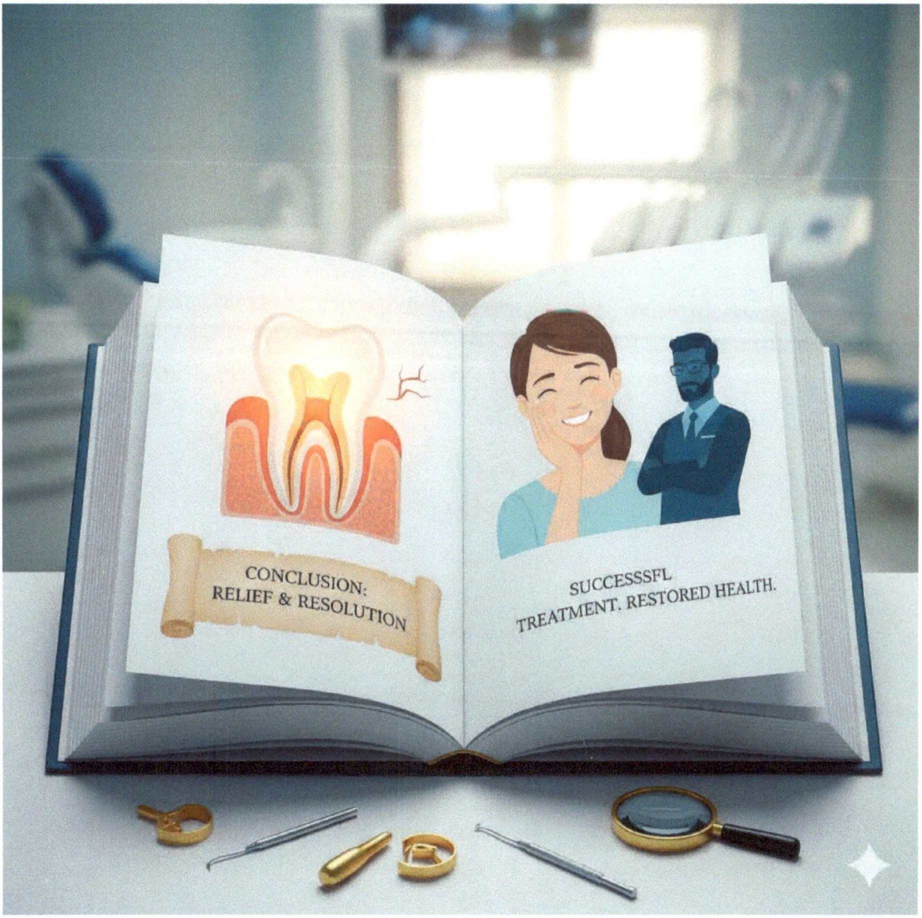
CONCLUSION:
RELIEF & RESOLUTION
SUCCESSSFL
TREATMENT. RESTORED HEALTH.

CONCLUSION

The prevalence of endodontic emergencies in dental practice is considerable, with over 80% of patients presenting with acute pain or related symptoms. This highlights the critical need for clinicians to possess comprehensive knowledge and proficiency in emergency management. Effective handling of such emergencies not only alleviates patient suffering but also strengthens trust in dental care providers.

A clinician's ability to make an accurate diagnosis forms the foundation of successful emergency management. This involves a thorough evaluation of the patient's medical and dental history, careful clinical examination, and the judicious use of diagnostic tests such as pulp vitality testing, radiographs, and percussion or palpation assessments. Correctly identifying the source and nature of the pain is essential to distinguish true endodontic emergencies from other orofacial conditions, ensuring that treatment is appropriately targeted and overtreatment is avoided.

Achieving profound local anaesthesia is a cornerstone of managing endodontic emergencies, particularly in cases of acute pulpitis or irreversible pulp inflammation, where pain control can be especially challenging. Clinicians should be skilled in advanced anaesthetic techniques, including intraosseous, intraligamentary, or supplemental buccal infiltrations, to ensure patient comfort during emergency interventions.

A sound treatment protocol is equally important. Immediate procedures, such as pulpotomy, pulpectomy, incision and drainage of abscesses, or extraction, must be guided by the diagnosis and aimed at rapid symptom relief. Prompt establishment of drainage, debridement of necrotic tissue, or removal of the irritant halts disease progression and provides immediate relief, often transforming a distressed patient into a reassured and grateful one.

Equally critical is the clinician's approach to patient care. Empathy, clear communication, and a calm, confident demeanor help control patient apprehension. Explaining the nature of the emergency, anticipated treatment outcomes, and post-procedural care reassures the patient, promotes compliance, and supports comprehensive healing.

Ultimately, the effective management of endodontic emergencies enhances the standard of dental care, improves patient outcomes, and bolsters the reputation of the profession. By continually updating clinical knowledge, refining diagnostic skills, and maintaining technical proficiency, dental practitioners ensure that even complex emergencies are managed competently and compassionately. This commitment represents both a professional obligation and a profound service to the community, advancing the image of dentistry as an essential and caring health profession.

BIBLIOGRAPHY

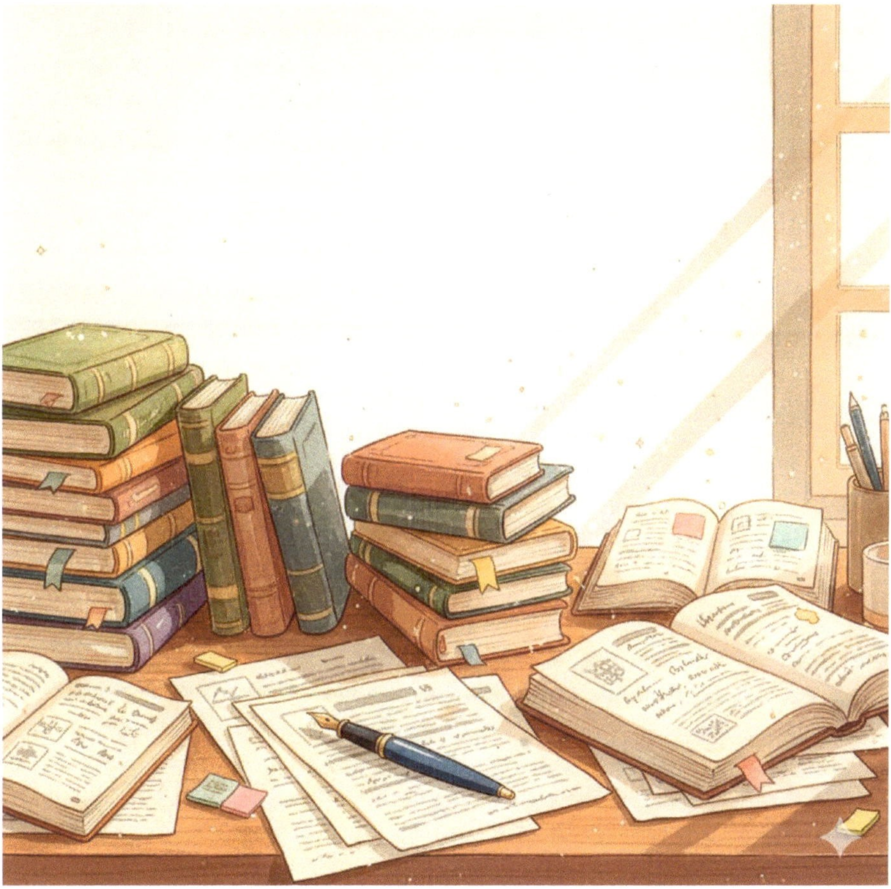

BIBLIOGRAPHY

1. Pratheebha C, Deepak S, Sandeep AH. Management of endodontic emergencies: A questionnaire survey. International journal of health sciences. 2022 Apr 16;6(S1):4958–72.
2. Abbott PV. Present status and future directions: Managing endodontic emergencies. International Endodontic Journal. 2022;55(S3):778–803.
3. Ali N, Srivastava V, SIngh A, Chauhan R. Endodontic Emergencies: An Overview. Asian Journal of Oral Health & Allied Science. 2018;8(1):31.
4. Torabinejad M, Wanlton R. Endodontic emergencies. In: Principles & Practices of Endodontics. 3rd ed. Saunders; 2002.
5. Dudeja PG, Dudeja KK, Srivastava D, Grover S. Microorganisms in Periradicular Tissues: Do they exist? A perennial controversy. J Oral Maxillofac Pathol. 2015;19(3):356–63.
6. Siqueira JF. Aetiology of Root Canal Treatment Failure: Why Well-Treated Teeth Can Fail. Int Endod J. 2001 Jan;34(1):1–10.
7. Omoigui S. The Biochemical Origin of Pain: The origin of all Pain is Inflammation and the Inflammatory Response. PART 2 of 3 –Inflammatory Profile of Pain Syndromes. Med Hypotheses. 2007;69(6):1169–78.
8. Torabinejad M, Fouad A, Shabahang S. Endodontics Principles and Practice. 6th ed. Elsevier; 2021.

9. B S, Gopikrishna V. Grossman's Endodontic Practice - 13th edition. 2014.
10. Tubiana M. [Wilhelm Conrad Röntgen and the discovery of X-rays]. Bull Acad Natl Med. 1996 Jan;180(1):97–108.
11. Specialty and Association Histories [Internet]. American Association of Endodontists. [cited 2025 Oct 16]. Available from: https://www.aae.org/specialty/about-aae/aae-history/specialty-association-histories/
12. Hargreaves KM, Berman LH. Cohen's Pathways of the Pulp. Mosby Elsevier; 2011. 952 p.
13. Bürklein S, Schäfer E, Donnermeyer D. Evaluation of a 3D-Printed Model as Complete Case Scenario in Undergraduate Dental Education-Diagnosis, Treatment Planning and Clinical Practice. Eur J Dent Educ. 2025 Apr 25;
14. Alkhattab OR, Alghamdi F, Abulhamael AM, Bakhsh A, Bahattab S, Kabbarah AJ, et al. Assessment of the Difference Between General Practitioners and Specialists in Antibiotic Prescription for Emergency Patients. South Eastern European Journal of Public Health. 2024 Sep 4;16–21.
15. Hanna SN, Perez Alfayate R, Prichard J. Vital Pulp Therapy an Insight Over the Available Literature and Future Expectations. Eur Endod J. 2020 Mar 1;5(1):46–53.
16. Koyuncuoglu G, Aren G. Clinical and radiographic evaluation of two different apexification protocols in traumatized immature permanent incisors. Ulus Travma Acil Cerrahi Derg. 2025 Jan;31(1):23–31.
17. Carrotte P. Endodontics: Part 3. Treatment of endodontic emergencies. Br Dent J. 2004 Sep 25;197(6):299–305.
18. Bachall J. Clinical Guide to Treating Endodontic Emergencies. Inside Dentistry. 2016;12(4):46–52.

19. Alhilou AM, Al-Moraissi EA, Bakhsh A, Christidis N, Näsman P. Pain after emergency treatments of symptomatic irreversible pulpitis and symptomatic apical periodontitis in the permanent dentition: a systematic review of randomized clinical trials. Front Oral Health. 2023 Oct 18;4:1147884.
20. Miglani S, Aggarwal V, Ahuja B. Dentin hypersensitivity: Recent trends in management. J Conserv Dent. 2010;13(4):218–24.
21. Holland GR, Narhi MN, Addy M, Gangarosa L, Orchardson R. Guidelines for the design and conduct of clinical trials on dentine hypersensitivity. J Clin Periodontol. 1997 Nov;24(11):808–13.
22. Addy M, Mostafa P, Newcombe RG. Dentine hypersensitivity: the distribution of recession, sensitivity and plaque. J Dent. 1987 Dec;15(6):242–8.
23. Raja SN, Carr DB, Cohen M, Finnerup NB, Flor H, Gibson S, et al. The Revised IASP definition of pain: concepts, challenges, and compromises. Pain. 2020 Sep 1;161(9):1976–82.
24. Davari A, Ataei E, Assarzadeh H. Dentin Hypersensitivity: Etiology, Diagnosis and Treatment; A Literature Review. J Dent (Shiraz). 2013 Sep;14(3):136–45.
25. Irvine JH. Root surface sensitivity: a review of aetiology and management. J N Z Soc Periodontol. 1988 Nov;(66):15–8.
26. Pashley DH. Dynamics of the pulpo-dentin complex. Crit Rev Oral Biol Med. 1996;7(2):104–33.
27. Braennstroem M, Astroem A. A study on the mechanism of pain elicited from the dentin. J Dent Res. 1964;43:619–25.
28. West N. The dentine hypersensitivity patient – a total management package. International Dental Journal. 2007;57(6 (Suppl 1)).

29. Canadian Advisory Board on Dentin Hypersensitivity. Consensus-based recommendations for the diagnosis and management of dentin hypersensitivity. J Can Dent Assoc. 2003 Apr;69(4):221–6.
30. Skallevold HE, Rokaya D, Khurshid Z, Zafar MS. Bioactive Glass Applications in Dentistry. Int J Mol Sci. 2019 Nov 27;20(23):5960.
31. Sionov RV, Tsavdaridou D, Aqawi M, Zaks B, Steinberg D, Shalish M. Tooth mousse containing casein phosphopeptide-amorphous calcium phosphate prevents biofilm formation of Streptococcus mutans. BMC Oral Health. 2021 Mar 19;21:136.
32. Imran F, Cooper PR, Ratnayake J, Ekambaram M, Mei ML. Potential Beneficial Effects of Hydroxyapatite Nanoparticles on Caries Lesions In Vitro—A Review of the Literature. Dentistry Journal. 2023 Feb;11(2):40.
33. Uraz A, Erol-Şii?mşek Ö, Pehlii?van S, Suludere Z, Bal B. The efficacy of 8% Arginine-CaCO3 applications on dentine hypersensitivity following periodontal therapy: A clinical and scanning electron microscopic study. Med Oral Patol Oral Cir Bucal. 2013 Mar;18(2):e298–305.
34. Sauro S, Carvalho RM, Ferracane J. The rise of advanced bioactive restorative materials: Are they redefining operative dentistry? Dental Materials. 2025 Nov 1;41(11):1411–29.
35. Lee BS, Chang CW, Chen WP, Lan WH, Lin CP. In vitro study of dentin hypersensitivity treated by Nd:YAP laser and bioglass. Dental Materials. 2005 Jun 1;21(6):511–9.
36. Peddi S, Hegde P, Reddy P, Barman A, Barik A, Dasgupta D, et al. Directed Self-Assembly of Magnetic Bioceramic Deep Inside Dentinal Tubules May Alleviate Dental Hypersensitivity. Advanced Science. 2025;12(39):e07664.

37. Bansode P, Pathlk S, Wavdhane M, Pandey A. The Hot Tooth. IOSR Journal of Dental and Medical Sciences. 2017;16(12):19–21.

38. Janani K, Teja KV, K H, Vasundhara KA, Jose J, Janani K, et al. Tackling Local Anesthetic Failure in Endodontics. In: Topics in Regional Anesthesia [Internet]. IntechOpen; 2021 [cited 2025 Oct 22]. Available from: https://www.intechopen.com/chapters/78272

39. Shoba J, Koshy M, Anirudhan S, Kalaichelvan T. Effective Strategies to Manage the Clinically Challenging Hot Tooth: A Review. Journal of Operative Dentistry & Endodontics. 2024 Apr 30;8(1):17–22.

40. Siqueira JF. Endodontic infections: Concepts, paradigms, and perspectives. Oral Surgery, Oral Medicine, Oral Pathology, Oral Radiology and Endodontics. 2002 Sep 1;94(3):281–93.

41. Williams BL, McCann GF, Schoenknecht FD. Bacteriology of dental abscesses of endodontic origin. J Clin Microbiol. 1983 Oct;18(4):770–4.

42. Rajendran A, Sivapathasundharam B. Shafer's Textbook of Oral Pathology. Elsevier Health Sciences; 2012. 1001 p.

43. Kakehashi S, Stanley HR, Fitzgerald RJ. The effects of surgical exposures of dental pulps in germ-free and conventional laboratory rats. Oral Surgery, Oral Medicine, Oral Pathology. 1965 Sep 1;20(3):340–9.

44. Naidorf IJ. Endodontic flare-ups: bacteriological and immunological mechanisms. J Endod. 1985 Nov;11(11):462–4.

45. Siqueira JF. Microbial causes of endodontic flare-ups. Int Endod J. 2003 Jul;36(7):453–63.

46. Hasan S, Singh K, Salati N. Cracked tooth syndrome: Overview of literature. Int J Appl Basic Med Res. 2015;5(3):164–8.

47. Cameron CE. The cracked tooth syndrome: additional findings. J Am Dent Assoc. 1976 Nov;93(5):971–5.

48. Banerji S, Mehta SB, Millar BJ. Cracked tooth syndrome. Part 1: aetiology and diagnosis. Br Dent J. 2010 May 22;208(10):459–63.

49. Diangelis AJ, Andreasen JO, Ebeleseder KA, Kenny DJ, Trope M, Sigurdsson A, et al. International Association of Dental Traumatology guidelines for the management of traumatic dental injuries: 1. Fractures and luxations of permanent teeth. Dent Traumatol. 2012 Feb;28(1):2–12.

50. Sharma B, Kaushal A. An overview of classification of traumatic injuries to tooth and its supporting structure. Glob J Res Anal. 2020 Jun;9(6).

51. Donnelly A, Foschi F, McCabe P, Duncan HF. Pulpotomy for treatment of complicated crown fractures in permanent teeth: A systematic review. Int Endod J. 2022 Apr;55(4):290–311.

52. Radwanski M, Caporossi C, Lukomska-Szymanska M, Luzi A, Sauro S. Complicated Crown Fracture of Permanent Incisors: A Conservative Treatment Case Report and a Narrative Review. Bioengineering (Basel). 2022 Sep 18;9(9):481.

53. Bajaj P, Chordiya R, Rudagi K, Patil N. Multidisciplinary approach to the management of complicated crown-root fracture: a case report. J Int Oral Health. 2015 Apr;7(4):88–91.

54. Lo Giudice R, Lizio A, Cervino G, Fabiana N, Francesco P, Ausiello P, et al. The Horizontal Root Fractures. Diagnosis, Clinical Management and Three-Year Follow-Up. Open Dent J. 2018;12:687–95.

55. Andreasen JO, Ahrensburg SS, Tsilingaridis G. Root fractures: the influence of type of healing and location of fracture on tooth

survival rates – an analysis of 492 cases. Dental Traumatology. 2012 Oct;28(5):404–9.

56. Abbott PV. Indications for root canal treatment following traumatic dental injuries to permanent teeth. Aust Dent J. 2023 Jun;68 Suppl 1:S123–40.
57. Myers GL. Evaluation and diagnosis of the traumatized dentition. Dent Traumatol. 2019 Dec;35(6):302–8.
58. Chen E, Abbott PV. Dental pulp testing: a review. Int J Dent. 2009;2009:365785.
59. Lima TFR, Dos Santos SL, Da Silva Fidalgo TK, Silva EJNL. Vitality Tests for Pulp Diagnosis of Traumatized Teeth: A Systematic Review. Journal of Endodontics. 2019 May;45(5):490–9.
60. Andreasen JO, Andreasen FM, Andersson L. Textbook and Color Atlas of Traumatic Injuries to the Teeth. EDUJ. 2019;6(4):279.
61. Alghaithy RA, Qualtrough AJE. Pulp sensibility and vitality tests for diagnosing pulpal health in permanent teeth: a critical review. Int Endod J. 2017 Feb;50(2):135–42.
62. Bourguignon C, Cohenca N, Lauridsen E, Flores MT, O'Connell AC, Day PF, et al. International Association of Dental Traumatology guidelines for the management of traumatic dental injuries: 1. Fractures and luxations. Dent Traumatol. 2020 Aug;36(4):314–30.
63. Sung L, Ku H, Shin Y, Swaid S, Kim D, Roh BD. Prognosis of Fragment Reattachment in Anterior Crown Fractures: A Retrospective Study. J Esthet Restor Dent. 2025 Jun;37(6):1557–66.
64. Shetty P, Padaru M, Bhat R. Minimal intervention treatment of a complicated crown fracture in a maxillary lateral incisor

by partial pulpotomy and fragment reattachment: A case report with a 10-year follow-up. World Acad Sci J. 2024 Jun 20;6(5):42.

65. Jain AK. Tuberculosis of the spine: a fresh look at an old disease. J Bone Joint Surg Br. 2010 Jul;92(7):905–13.

66. Levin L, Day PF, Hicks L, O'Connell A, Fouad AF, Bourguignon C, et al. International Association of Dental Traumatology guidelines for the management of traumatic dental injuries: General introduction. Dental Traumatology. 2020 Aug;36(4):309–13.

67. Murray PE, Windsor Lj, Smyth Tw, Hafez Aa, Cox CF. A Nalysis of P Ulpal R Eactions to R Estorative P Rocedures, M Aterials, P Ulp C Apping, And F Uture T Herapies. Critical Reviews in Oral Biology & Medicine. 2002 Nov;13(6):509–20.

68. Magnusson BO, Sundell SO. Stepwise excavation of deep carious lesions in primary molars. J Int Assoc Dent Child. 1977 Dec;8(2):36–40.

69. Leksell E, Ridell K, Cvek M, Mejàre I. Pulp exposure after stepwise versus direct complete excavation of deep carious lesions in young posterior permanent teeth. Endod Dent Traumatol. 1996 Aug;12(4):192–6.

70. Wittrock JW, Morrant GA, Davies EH. A study of temperature changes during removal of amalgam restorations. J Prosthet Dent. 1975 Aug;34(2):179–86.

71. Seeburrun, R. (2004). How might Operative Dentistry be a Threat to the Pulp?. Trinity Student Medical Journal , 5(1), Page 50–54.

72. Walton R, Fouad A. Endodontic interappointment flare-ups: a prospective study of incidence and related factors. J Endod. 1992 Apr;18(4):172–7.

73. Siqueira JF. Microbial causes of endodontic flare-ups. Int Endod J. 2003 Jul;36(7):453–63.

74. Pak JG, White SN. Pain prevalence and severity before, during, and after root canal treatment: a systematic review. J Endod. 2011 Apr;37(4):429–38.

75. Mor C, Rotstein I, Friedman S. Incidence of interappointment emergency associated with endodontic therapy. J Endod. 1992 Oct;18(10):509–11.

76. Tsesis I, Faivishevsky V, Fuss Z, Zukerman O. Flare-ups after Endodontic Treatment: A Meta-analysis of Literature. Journal of Endodontics. 2008 Oct;34(10):1177–81.

77. Di Spirito F, Scelza G, Fornara R, Giordano F, Rosa D, Amato A. Post-Operative Endodontic Pain Management: An Overview of Systematic Reviews on Post-Operatively Administered Oral Medications and Integrated Evidence-Based Clinical Recommendations. Healthcare (Basel). 2022 Apr 19;10(5):760.

78. Sadaf D, Ahmad MZ. Factors associated with postoperative pain in endodontic therapy. Int J Biomed Sci. 2014 Dec;10(4):243–7.

79. Pak JG, White SN. Pain prevalence and severity before, during, and after root canal treatment: a systematic review. J Endod. 2011 Apr;37(4):429–38.

80. Torabinejad M, Walton RE. Managing Endodontic Emergencis. The Journal of the American Dental Association. 1991 May;122(5):99–103.

81. Jayakodi H, Kailasam S, Kumaravadivel K, Thangavelu B, Mathew S. Clinical and pharmacological management of endodontic flare-up. J Pharm Bioallied Sci. 2012 Aug;4(Suppl 2):S294-298.

82. Jakovljevic A, Andric M. Human Cytomegalovirus and Epstein-Barr Virus in Etiopathogenesis of Apical Periodontitis: A Systematic Review. Journal of Endodontics. 2014 Jan;40(1):6–15.
83. Graunaite I, Lodiene G, Maciulskiene V. Pathogenesis of apical periodontitis: a literature review. J Oral Maxillofac Res. 2012 Jan 1;2(4):e1.
84. Torabinejad M, Bakland LK. Immunopathogenesis of chronic periapical lesions. A review. Oral Surg Oral Med Oral Pathol. 1978 Nov;46(5):685–99.
85. Siqueira JF, Barnett F. Interappointment pain: mechanisms, diagnosis, and treatment. Endodontic Topics. 2004 Mar;7(1):93–109.
86. Sipavičiūtė E, Manelienė R. Pain and flare-up after endodontic treatment procedures. Stomatologija. 2014;16(1):25–30.
87. Ehrmann EH, Messer HH, Adams GG. The relationship of intracanal medicaments to postoperative pain in endodontics. Int Endod J. 2003 Dec;36(12):868–75.
88. Ehrmann EH, Messer HH, Adams GG. The relationship of intracanal medicaments to postoperative pain in endodontics. Int Endod J. 2003 Dec;36(12):868–75.
89. Rogers MJ, Johnson BR, Remeikis NA, BeGole EA. Comparison of effect of intracanal use of ketorolac tromethamine and dexamethasone with oral ibuprofen on post treatment endodontic pain. J Endod. 1999 May;25(5):381–4.
90. Negm MM. Intracanal use of a corticosteroid-antibiotic compound for the management of posttreatment endodontic pain. Oral Surg Oral Med Oral Pathol Oral Radiol Endod. 2001 Oct;92(4):435–9.
91. Pozzi A, Gallelli L. Pain management for dentists: the role of ibuprofen. Ann Stomatol (Roma). 2011 Jul;2(3-4 Suppl):3–24.

92. Sethi P, Agarwal M, Chourasia HR, Singh MP. Effect of single dose pretreatment analgesia with three different analgesics on postoperative endodontic pain: A randomized clinical trial. J Conserv Dent. 2014 Nov;17(6):517–21.

93. Curtis P, Gartman LA, Green DB. Utilization of ketorolac tromethamine for control of severe odontogenic pain. Journal of Endodontics. 1994 Sep;20(9):457–9.

94. Yadav RK, Yadav HK, Chandra A, Yadav S, Verma P, Shakya VK. Accidental aspiration/ingestion of foreign bodies in dentistry: A clinical and legal perspective. Natl J Maxillofac Surg. 2015;6(2):144–51.

95. Webb WA. Management of foreign bodies of the upper gastrointestinal tract. Gastroenterology. 1988 Jan;94(1):204–16.

96. Tamura N, Nakajima T, Matsumoto S, Ohyama T, Ohashi Y. Foreign bodies of dental origin in the air and food passages. International Journal of Oral and Maxillofacial Surgery. 1986 Dec;15(6):739–51.

97. Susini G, Pommel L, Camps J. Accidental ingestion and aspiration of root canal instruments and other dental foreign bodies in a French population. Int Endodontic J. 2007 Aug;40(8):585–9.

98. Tiwana KK, Morton T, Tiwana PS. Aspiration and ingestion in dental practice: a 10-year institutional review. J Am Dent Assoc. 2004 Sep;135(9):1287–91.

99. Govila CP. Accidental swallowing of an endodontic instrument. Oral Surgery, Oral Medicine, Oral Pathology. 1979 Sep;48(3):269–71.

100. Sharma S, Sonali, Asusa, Udhey C, Kour P, Chauhan M. A literature review on complications and management of

use sodium hypochlorite in endodontics. IJCE. 2021 Dec 28;6(4):191–3.

101. Crane AB. A practicable root canal technique. Philadelphia: Lea & Febinger; 1920.

102. Rahimi S, Janani M, Lotfi M, Shahi S, Aghbali A, Vahid Pakdel M, et al. A review of antibacterial agents in endodontic treatment. Iran Endod J. 2014;9(3):161–8.

103. Sreelakshmi SB, Anjaneyulu K, Geetha RV, Modification and Methods to Improve the Efficiency of Sodium Hypochlorite as A Root Canal Irrigant, J Res Med Dent Sci, 2020, 8 (7): 308-317.

104. Mohammadi Z. Sodium hypochlorite in endodontics: an update review. Int Dent J. 2008 Dec;58(6):329–41.

105. Lecturer, Nitte (Deemed to be University), AB Shetty Memorial Institute Of Dental Sciences(ABSMIDS), Department of Conservative Dentistry and Endodontics, Bhat R. Insight on the Use and Abuse of Sodium Hypochlorite in Endodontics: A Review. IJDOS. 2021 Aug 19;4028–31.

106. Vivekananda Pai AR. Factors influencing the occurrence and progress of sodium hypochlorite accident: A narrative and update review. J Conserv Dent. 2023;26(1):3–11.

107. Gamal-AbdelNaser A, Elnaggar A, Mekawy M, Boshra G, Ghareeb N. Sodium hypochlorite accident—complications, management and potential prevention: a report of three cases. Front Oral Maxillofac Med. 2025 Jun;7:12–12.

108. Udhey C, Kour P, Chauhan M, Sharma S. A literature review on complications and management of use sodium hypochlorite in endodontics. IP Indian J. Conserv. Endod. 2021;6:191-3.

109. Perotti S, Bin P, Cecchi R. Hypochlorite accident during wndodontic therapy with nerve damage - A case report. Acta Biomed. 2018 Mar 27;89(1):104–8.

110. Nasiri K, Wrbas KT. Management of sodium hypochlorite accident in root canal treatment. J Dent Sci. 2023 Apr;18(2):945–6.

111. Ho JPTF, van Riet TCT, Afrian Y, Sem KTHCJ, Spijker R, de Lange J, et al. Adverse effects following dental local anesthesia: a literature review. J Dent Anesth Pain Med. 2021 Dec;21(6):507–25.

112. Khalifeh B, Simonian K, Houmani M, El-Outa A, Khalil W. Trismus Following Inferior Alveolar Nerve Block: A Case Report. Cureus. 2024 Nov;16(11):e73394.

113. Bassam S, El-Ahmar R, Salloum S, Ayoub S. Endodontic postoperative flare-up: An update. Saudi Dent J. 2021 Nov;33(7):386–94.

114. Basil Yousif Alamassi. Endodontic Postoperative Pain: Etiology and Related Factors – An Update. International Journal of Dental Sciences and Research. Vol. 5, No. 2, 2017, pp 13-21.

115. Vivekananda Pai A, Shrikrishna S, Shah N. Surgical management of overfilled gutta-percha and root capping with mineral trioxide aggregate in a young patient. J Interdiscip Dentistry. 2014;4(3):148.

116. Malagnino VA, Pappalardo A, Plotino G, Carlesi T. The fate of overfilling in root canal treatments with long-term follow-up: a case series. Restor Dent Endod. 2021 May;46(2):e27.

117. Almas B, Rao HM, Prasad B. Vertical Root Fractures – A Review. In [cited 2025 Nov 8]. Available from: https://www.semanticscholar. org/paper/Vertical-Root-Fractures-

%E2%80%93-A-Review-Almas-Rao/082b8b2fbeaac4fc210caef38e69679ce16414ca

118. Alsani A, Balhaddad A, Nazir MA. Vertical root fracture: a case report and review of the literature. Giornale Italiano di Endodonzia. 2017 Jun 30;31(1):21–8.

119. Jacob G, Niranjan NT, Babannavar R. Management of Complicated Crown Fracture by Partial Pulpotomy & Fragment Reattachment: A Case Report. RGUHS Journal of Dental Sciences. 2022;14(4).

www.ingramcontent.com/pod-product-compliance
Lightning Source LLC
LaVergne TN
LVHW051134210926
848482LV00006B/308
* 9 7 9 8 9 0 3 4 2 7 5 3 6 *